Better

Better

A SURGEON'S NOTES
ON PERFORMANCE

Atul Gawande

P

PROFILE BOOKS

First published in Great Britain in 2007 by
PROFILE BOOKS LTD
3A Exmouth House
Pine Street
London EC1R 0JH
www.profilebooks.com

First published in the United States of America in 2007 by
Metropolitan Books

Several of these chapters have appeared, in different form,
in the *New Yorker* and the *New England Journal of Medicine*

1 3 5 7 9 10 8 6 4 2

Designed by Meryl Sussman Lavavi

Printed and bound in Great Britain by
Clays, Bungay, Suffolk

A CIP catalogue record for this book is available from the British Library.

ISBN 978 1 86197 897 4

The paper this book is printed on is certified by the © 1996 Forest Stewardship
Council A.C. (FSC). It is ancient-forest friendly. The printer holds FSC chain of custody
SGS-COC-2061

FSC
Mixed Sources
Product group from well-managed
forests and other controlled sources

Cert no. SGS-COC-2061
www.fsc.org
© 1996 Forest Stewardship Council

For my parents and sister

Contents

Better

Introduction

Several years ago, in my final year of medical school, I took care of a patient who has stuck in my mind. I was on an internal medicine rotation, my last rotation before graduating. The senior resident had assigned me primary responsibility for three or four patients. One was a wrinkled, seventy-something-year-old Portuguese woman who had been admitted because—I'll use the technical term here—she didn't feel too good. Her body ached. She had become tired all the time. She had a cough. She had no fever. Her pulse and blood pressure were fine. But some laboratory tests revealed her white blood cell count was abnormally high. A chest X-ray showed a possible pneumonia—maybe it was, maybe it wasn't. So her internist admitted her to the hospital, and now she was under my care. I took sputum and blood cultures and, following the internist's instructions, started her on an antibiotic for this possible pneumonia. I went to see her twice each day for the next several days. I checked her vital signs, listened to her lungs, looked up her labs. Each day, she stayed more or less the same. She had a cough. She had no fever. She just didn't feel good. We'd give her antibiotics and wait her out, I figured. She'd be fine.

One morning on seven o'clock rounds, she complained of insomnia and having sweats overnight. We checked the vitals sheets. She still had no fever. Her blood pressure was normal. Her heart rate was running maybe slightly faster than before. But that was all. Keep a close eye on her, the senior resident told me. Of course, I said, though nothing we'd seen seemed remarkably different from previous mornings. I made a silent plan to see her at midday, around lunchtime. The senior resident, however, went back to check on her himself twice that morning.

It is this little act that I have often thought about since. It was a small thing, a tiny act of conscientiousness. He had seen something about her that worried him. He had also taken the measure of me on morning rounds. And what he saw was a fourth-year student, with a residency spot already lined up in general surgery, on his last rotation of medical school. Did he trust me? No, he did not. So he checked on her himself.

That was not a two-second matter, either. She was up on the fourteenth floor of the hospital. Our morning teaching conferences, the cafeteria, all the other places we had to be that day were on the bottom two floors. The elevators were notoriously slow. The senior resident was supposed to run one of those teaching conferences. He could have waited for a nurse to let him know if a problem arose, as most doctors would. He could have told a junior resident to see the patient. But he didn't. He made himself go up.

The first time he did, he found she had a fever of 102 degrees and needed the oxygen flow through her nasal prongs increased. The second time, he found her blood pressure had dropped and the nurses had switched her oxygen to a face mask, and he transferred her to the intensive care unit. By the time I had a clue about what was going on, he already had her under treatment—with new antibiotics, intravenous fluids, medications to support her blood pressure—for what was developing into septic shock from a resistant, fulminant pneumonia. Because he checked on her, she survived. Indeed, because he did, her course was beautiful. She never needed to be put on a ventilator. The fevers stopped in twenty-four hours. She got home in three days.

WHAT DOES IT take to be good at something in which failure is so easy, so effortless? When I was a student and then a resident, my deepest concern was to become competent. But what that senior resident had displayed that day was more than competence—he grasped not just how a pneumonia generally evolves and is properly treated but also the particulars of how to catch and fight one in that specific patient, in that specific moment, with the specific resources and people he had at hand.

People often look to great athletes for lessons about performance. And for a surgeon like me, athletes do indeed have lessons to teach—about the value of perseverance, of hard work and practice, of precision. But success in medicine has dimensions that cannot be found on a playing field. For one, lives are on the line. Our decisions and omissions are therefore moral in nature. We also face daunting expectations. In medicine, our task is to cope with illness and to enable every human being to lead a life as long and free of frailty as science will allow. The steps are often uncertain. The knowledge to be mastered is both vast and incomplete. Yet we are expected to act with swiftness and consistency, even when the task requires marshaling hundreds of people—from laboratory technicians to the nurses on each change of shift to the engineers who keep the oxygen supply system working—for the care of a single person. We are also expected to do our work humanely, with gentleness and concern. It's not only the stakes but also the complexity of performance in medicine that makes it so interesting and, at the same time, so unsettling.

Recently, I took care of a patient with breast cancer. Virginia Magboo was sixty-four years old, an English teacher, and she'd noticed a pebblelike lump in her breast. A needle biopsy revealed the diagnosis. The cancer was small—three-quarters of an inch in diameter. She considered her options and decided on breast-conserving treatment—I'd do a wide excision of the lump as well as what's called a sentinel lymph node biopsy to make sure the cancer hadn't spread to the lymph nodes. Radiation would follow.

The operation was not going to be difficult or especially hazardous, but the team had to be meticulous about every step. On the day of surgery, before bringing her to the operating room, the anesthesiologist double-checked that it was safe to proceed. She reviewed Magboo's medical history and medications, looked at her labs in the computer and at her EKG. She made sure that the patient had not had anything to eat for at least six hours and had her open her mouth to note any loose teeth that could fall out or dentures that should be removed. A nurse checked the patient's name band to make sure we had the right person; verified her drug allergies with her, confirmed that the procedure listed on her consent form was the one she expected. The nurse also looked for contact lenses that shouldn't be left in and for jewelry that could constrict a finger or snag on something. I made a mark with a felt-tip pen over the precise spot where Magboo felt the lump, so there would be no mistaking the correct location. Early in the morning before her surgery, she had also had a small amount of radioactive tracer injected near her breast lump, in preparation for the sentinel lymph node biopsy. I now used a hand-held Geiger counter to locate where the tracer had flowed, and confirmed that the counts were strong enough to indicate which lymph node was the "hot" one that needed to be excised. Meanwhile, in the operating room, two nurses made sure the room had been thoroughly cleaned after the previous procedure and that we had all the equipment we needed. There is a sticker on the surgical instrument kit that turns brown if the kit has been heat-sterilized and they confirmed that the sticker had turned. A technician removed the electrocautery machine and replaced it with another one after a question was raised about how it was functioning. Everything was checked and cross-checked. Magboo and the team were ready.

By two o'clock I had finished with the procedures for my

patients before her and I was ready too. Then I got a phone call.

Her case was being delayed, a woman from the OR control desk told me.

Why? I asked.

The recovery room was full. So three operating rooms were unable to bring their patients out, and all further procedures were halted until the recovery room opened up.

OK. No problem. This happens once in a while. We'll wait. By four o'clock, however, Magboo still had not been taken in. I called down to the OR desk to find out what was going on.

The recovery room had opened up, I was told, but Magboo was getting bumped for a patient with a ruptured aortic aneurysm coming down from the emergency room. The staff would work on getting us another OR.

I explained the situation to Magboo, lying on her stretcher in the preoperative holding area, and apologized. Shouldn't be too much longer, I told her. She was philosophical. What will be will be, she said. She tried to sleep to make the time pass more quickly but kept waking up. Each time she awoke, nothing had changed.

At six o'clock I called again and spoke to the OR desk manager. They had a room for me, he said, but no nurses. After five o'clock, there are only enough nurses available to cover seventeen of our forty-two operating rooms. And twenty-three cases were going at that moment—he'd already made nurses in four rooms do mandatory overtime and could not make any more. There was no way to fit another patient in.

Well, when did he see Magboo going?

"She may not be going at all," he said. After seven, he pointed out, he'd have nurses for only nine rooms; after eleven, he could run at most five. And Magboo was not the only patient waiting. "She will likely have to be canceled," he said. Cancel her? How could we cancel her?

I went down to the control desk in person. One surgeon was already there ahead of me lobbying the anesthesiologist in charge. A second was yelling into the OR manager's ear on the phone. Each of us wanted an operating room and there would not be enough to go around. A patient had a lung cancer that needed to be removed. Another patient had a mass in his neck that needed to be biopsied. "My case is quick," one surgeon argued. "My patient cannot wait," said another. Operating rooms were offered for the next day and none of us wanted to take one. We each had other patients already scheduled who would themselves have to be canceled to make room. And what was to keep this mess from happening all over again tomorrow, anyway?

I tried to make my case for Magboo. She had a breast cancer. It needed to be taken out. This had to happen sooner rather than later. The radioactive tracer, injected more than eight hours ago, was dissipating by the hour. Postponing her operation would mean she would have to undergo a second injection of a radioactive tracer—a doubling of her radiation exposure—just because an OR could not be found for her. That would be unconscionable, I said.

No one, however, would make any promises.

*   *   *

THIS IS A book about performance in medicine. As a doctor, you go into this work thinking it is all a matter of canny diagnosis, technical prowess, and some ability to empathize with people. But it is not, you soon find out. In medicine, as in any profession, we must grapple with systems, resources, circumstances, people—and our own shortcomings, as well. We face obstacles of seemingly unending variety. Yet somehow we must advance, we must refine, we must improve. How we have and how we do is my subject here.

The sections of this book examine three core requirements for success in medicine—or in any endeavor that involves risk and responsibility. The first is diligence, the necessity of giving sufficient attention to detail to avoid error and prevail against obstacles. Diligence seems an easy and minor virtue. (You just pay attention, right?) But it is neither. Diligence is both central to performance and fiendishly hard, as I show through three stories: one about the effort to ensure doctors and nurses simply wash their hands; one about the care of the wounded soldiers in Iraq and Afghanistan; and one about the Herculean effort to eradicate polio from the globe.

The second challenge is to do right. Medicine is a fundamentally human profession. It is therefore forever troubled by human failings, failings like avarice, arrogance, insecurity, misunderstanding. In this section I consider some of our most uncomfortable questions—such as how much doctors should be paid, and what we owe patients when we make mistakes. I tell the stories of four doctors and a nurse who have gone against medical ethics codes and participated in executions of prisoners. I puzzle over how we know when we should keep fighting for a sick patient and when we should stop.

The third requirement for success is ingenuity—thinking anew. Ingenuity is often misunderstood. It is not a matter of superior intelligence but of character. It demands more than anything a willingness to recognize failure, to not paper over the cracks, and to change. It arises from deliberate, even obsessive, reflection on failure and a constant searching for new solutions. These are difficult traits to foster—but they are far from impossible ones. Here I tell the stories of people in everyday medicine who have, through ingenuity, transformed medical care—for example, the way babies are delivered and the way an incurable disease like cystic fibrosis is fought—and I examine how more of us can do the same.

Betterment is a perpetual labor. The world is chaotic, disorganized, and vexing, and medicine is nowhere spared that reality. To complicate matters, we in medicine are also only humans ourselves. We are distractible, weak, and given to our own concerns. Yet still, to live as a doctor is to live so that one's life is bound up in others' and in science and in the messy, complicated connection between the two. It is to live a life of responsibility. The question, then, is not whether one accepts the responsibility. Just by doing this work, one has. The question is, having accepted the responsibility, how one does such work well.

VIRGINIA MAGBOO LAY waiting, anxious and hungry, in a windowless, silent, white-lit holding area for still two hours more.

The minutes ticked, ticked, ticked. At times, in medicine, you feel you are inside a colossal and impossibly complex machine whose gears will turn for you only according to their own arbitrary rhythm. The notion that human caring, the effort to do better for people, might make a difference can seem hopelessly naïve. But it isn't.

Magboo asked me if there was any real prospect of her having her operation that night. The likelihood, I said, had become exceedingly small. But I couldn't bring myself to send her home, and I asked her to hang on with me. Then, just before eight o'clock, I got a text message on my pager. "We can bring your patient back to room 29," the display read. Two nurses, it turned out, had seen how backed up the ORs had gotten and, although they could easily have gone home, they volunteered to stay late. "I didn't really have anything else going on anyway," one demurred when I spoke to her. When you make an effort, you find sometimes you are not the only one willing to do so.

Eleven minutes after I got the page, Magboo was on the operating table, a sedative going into her arm. Her skin was cleansed. Her body was draped. The breast cancer came out without difficulty. Her lymph nodes proved to be free of metastasis. And she was done. She woke up calmly as we put on the dressing. I saw her gazing upward at the operating light above her.

"The light looks like seashells," she said.

PART I

Diligence

On Washing Hands

One ordinary December day, I took a tour of my hospital with Deborah Yokoe, an infectious disease specialist, and Susan Marino, a microbiologist. They work in our hospital's infection-control unit. Their full-time job, and that of three others in the unit, is to stop the spread of infection in the hospital. This is not flashy work, and they are not flashy people. Yokoe is forty-five years old, gentle voiced, and dimpled. She wears sneakers at work. Marino is in her fifties and reserved by nature. But they have coped with influenza epidemics, Legionnaires' disease, fatal bacterial meningitis, and, just a few months before, a case that, according to the patient's brain-biopsy results, might have been Creutzfeld-Jakob disease—a nightmare, not only because it is incurable and fatal but also because the infectious agent that causes it, known as a prion, cannot be killed by usual heat-sterilization procedures. By the time the results came back, the neurosurgeon's brain-biopsy instruments might have transferred the disease to other patients, but infection-control team members tracked the instruments down in time and had them chemically sterilized. Yokoe and Marino have seen measles, the plague, and rabbit fever (which is caused by a bacterium that is extraordinarily contagious in hospital laboratories and feared as a bioterrorist weapon). They once instigated a nationwide recall of frozen strawberries, having traced a hepatitis A outbreak to a batch served at an ice cream social. Recently at large in the hospital, they told me, have been a rotavirus, a Norwalk virus, several strains of *Pseudomonas* bacteria, a superresistant *Klebsiella*, and the ubiquitous scourges of modern hospitals—resistant *Staphylococcus aureus* and *Enterococcus faecalis*, which are a frequent cause of pneumonias, wound infections, and bloodstream infections.

Each year, according to the U.S. Centers for Disease Control, two million Americans acquire an infection while they are in the hospital. Ninety thousand die of that infection. The hardest part of the infection-control team's job, Yokoe says, is not coping with the variety of contagions they encounter or the panic that sometimes occurs among patients and staff. Instead, their greatest difficulty is getting clinicians like me to do the one thing that consistently halts the spread of infections: wash our hands.

There isn't much they haven't tried. Walking about the surgical floors where I admit my patients, Yokoe and Marino showed me the admonishing signs they have posted, the sinks they have repositioned, the new ones they have installed. They have made some sinks automated. They have bought special five-thousand-dollar "precaution carts" that store everything for washing up, gloving, and gowning in one ergonomic, portable, and aesthetically pleasing package. They have given away free movie tickets to the hospital units with the best compliance. They have issued hygiene report cards. Yet still, we have not mended our ways. Our hospital's statistics show what studies everywhere else have shown—that we doctors and nurses wash our hands one-third to one-half as often as we are supposed to. Having shaken hands with a sniffling patient, pulled a sticky dressing off someone's wound, pressed a stethoscope against a sweating chest, most of us do little more than wipe our hands on our white coats and move on—to see the next patient, to scribble a note in the chart, to grab some lunch.

This is, embarassingly, nothing new. In 1847, at the age of twenty-eight, the Viennese obstetrician Ignac Semmelweis famously deduced that, by not washing their hands consistently or well enough, doctors were themselves to blame for childbed fever. Childbed fever, also known as puerperal fever, was the leading cause of maternal death in childbirth in the era before antibiotics (and before the recognition that germs are the agents of infectious disease). It is a bacterial infection—most commonly caused by *Streptococcus*, the same bacteria that causes strep throat—that ascends through the vagina to the uterus after childbirth. Out of three thousand mothers who delivered babies at the hospital where Semmelweis worked, six hundred or more died of the disease each year—a horrifying 20 percent maternal death rate. Of mothers delivering at home, only 1 percent died. Semmelweis concluded that doctors themselves were carrying the disease between patients, and he mandated that every doctor and nurse on his ward scrub with a nail brush and chlorine between patients. The puerperal death rate immediately fell to 1 percent—incontrovertible proof, it would seem, that he was right. Yet elsewhere, doctors' practices did not change. Some colleagues were even offended by his claims; it was impossible to them that doctors could be killing their patients. Far from being hailed, Semmelweis was ultimately dismissed from his job.

Semmelweis's story has come down to us as Exhibit A in the case for the obstinacy and blindness of physicians. But the story was more complicated. The trouble was partly that nineteenth-century physicians faced multiple, seemingly equally powerful explanations for puerperal fever. There was, for example, a strong belief that miasmas of the air in hospitals were the cause. And Semmelweis strangely refused to either publish an explanation of the logic behind his theory or prove it with a convincing experiment in animals. Instead, he took the calls for proof as a personal insult and attacked his detractors viciously.

"You, Herr Professor, have been a partner in this massacre," he wrote to one University of Vienna obstetrician who questioned his theory. To a colleague in Wurzburg he wrote, "Should you, Herr Hofrath, without having disproved my doctrine, continue to teach your pupils [against it], I declare before God and the world that you are a murderer and the 'History of Childbed Fever' would not be unjust to you if it memorialized you as a medical Nero." His own staff turned against him. In Pest, where he relocated after losing his post in

Vienna, he would stand next to the sink and berate anyone who forgot to scrub his or her hands. People began to purposely evade, sometimes even sabotage, his hand-washing regimen. Semmelweis was a genius, but he was also a lunatic, and that made him a failed genius. It was another twenty years before Joseph Lister offered his clearer, more persuasive, and more respectful plea for antisepsis in surgery in the British medical journal *Lancet*.

One hundred and forty years of doctors' plagues later, however, you have to wonder whether what's needed to stop them is precisely a lunatic. Consider what Yokoe and Marino are up against. No part of human skin is spared from bacteria. Bacterial counts on the hands range from five thousand to five million colony-forming units per square centimeter. The hair, underarms, and groin harbor greater concentrations. On the hands, deep skin crevices trap 10 to 20 percent of the flora, making removal difficult, even with scrubbing, and sterilization impossible. The worst place is under the fingernails. Hence the recent CDC guidelines requiring hospital personnel to keep their nails trimmed to less than a quarter of an inch and to remove artificial nails.

Plain soaps do, at best, a middling job of disinfecting. Their detergents remove loose dirt and grime, but fifteen seconds of washing reduces bacterial counts by only about an order of magnitude. Semmelweis recognized that ordinary soap was not enough and used a chlorine solution to achieve disinfection. Today's antibacterial soaps contain chemicals such as chlorhexidine to disrupt microbial membranes and proteins. Even with the right soap, however, proper hand washing requires a strict procedure. First, you must remove your watch, rings, and other jewelry (which are notorious for trapping bacteria). Next, you wet your hands in warm tap water. Dispense the soap and lather all surfaces, including the lower one-third of the arms, for the full duration recommended by the manufacturer (usually fifteen to thirty seconds). Rinse off for thirty full seconds. Dry completely with a clean, disposable towel. Then use the towel to turn the tap off. Repeat after any new contact with a patient.

Almost no one adheres to this procedure. It seems impossible. On morning rounds, our residents check in on twenty patients in an hour. The nurses in our intensive care units typically have a similar number of contacts with patients requiring hand washing in between. Even if you get the whole cleansing process down to a minute per patient, that's still a third of staff time spent just washing hands. Such frequent hand washing can also irritate the skin, which can produce a dermatitis, which itself increases bacterial counts.

Less irritating than soap, alcohol rinses and gels have been in use in Europe for almost two decades but for some reason only recently caught on in the United States. They take far less time to use—only about fifteen seconds or so to rub a gel over the hands and fingers and let it air-dry. Dispensers can be put at the bedside more easily than a sink. And at alcohol concentrations of 50 to 95 percent, they are more effective at killing organisms, too. (Interestingly, pure alcohol is not as effective—at least some water is required to denature microbial proteins.)

Still, it took Yokoe over a year to get our staff to accept the 60 percent alcohol gel we have recently adopted. Its introduction was first blocked because of the staff's fears that it would produce noxious building air. (It didn't.) Next came worries that, despite evidence to the contrary, it would be more irritating to the skin. So a product with aloe was brought in. People complained about the smell. So the aloe was taken out. Then some of the nursing staff refused to use the gel after rumors spread that it would reduce fertility. The rumors died only after the infection-control unit circulated evidence that the alcohol is not systemically absorbed and a hospital fertility specialist endorsed the use of the gel.

With the gel finally in wide use, the compliance rates for proper hand hygiene improved substantially: from around 40 percent to 70 percent. But—and this is the troubling finding—hospital infection rates did not drop one iota. Our 70 percent compliance just wasn't good enough. If 30 percent of the time people didn't wash their hands, that still left plenty of opportunity to keep transmitting infections. Indeed, the rates of resistant *Staphylococcus* and *Enterococcus* infections continued to rise. Yokoe receives the daily tabulations. I checked with her one day not long ago, and sixty-three of our seven hundred hospital patients were colonized or infected with MRSA (the shorthand for methicillin-resistant *Staphylococcus aureus*) and another twenty-two had acquired VRE (vancomycin-resistant *Enterococcus*)—unfortunately, typical rates of infection for American hospitals.

Rising infection rates from superresistant bacteria have become the norm around the world. The first outbreak of VRE did not occur until 1988, when a renal dialysis unit in England became infested. By 1990, the bacteria had been carried abroad, and four in one thousand American ICU patients had become infected. By 1997, a stunning 23 percent of ICU patients were infected. When the virus for SARS—severe acute respiratory syndrome—appeared in China in 2003 and spread within weeks to almost ten thousand people in two dozen countries across the world (10 percent of whom were killed), the primary vector for transmission was the hands of health care workers. What will happen if (or rather, when) an even more dangerous organism appears—avian flu, say, or a new, more virulent bacteria? "It will be a disaster," Yokoe says.

Anything short of a Semmelweis-like obsession with hand washing has begun to seem inadequate. Yokoe, Marino, and their colleagues have now resorted to doing random spot checks on the floors. On a surgical intensive care unit, they showed me what they do. They walk in unannounced. They go directly into patients' rooms. They check for unattended spills, toilets that have not been cleaned, faucets that drip, empty gel dispensers, overflowing needle boxes, inadequate supplies of gloves and gowns. They check whether the nurses are wearing gloves when they handle patients' wound dressings and catheters, which are ready portals for infection. And of course, they watch to see whether everyone is washing up before patient contact. Neither hesitates to confront people, though they try to be gentle about it. ("Did you forget to gel your hands?" is a favored line.) Staff members have come to recognize them. I watched a gloved and gowned nurse come out of a patient's room, pick up the patient's chart (which is not supposed to be touched by dirty hands), see Marino, and immediately stop short. "I didn't touch anything in the room! I'm clean!" she blurted out.

Yokoe and Marino hate this aspect of the job. They don't want to be infection cops. It's no fun, and it's not necessarily effective, either. With twelve patient floors and four different patient pods per floor, they can't stand watch the way Semmelweis did, scowling over the lone sink on his unit. And they risk having the staff revolt as his staff did against him. But what other options remain? I flipped through back issues of the *Journal of Hospital Infection* and *Infection Control and Hospital Epidemiology*, two leading journals in the field, and the articles are a sad litany of failed experiments to change our contaminating ways. The great hoped-for solution has been a soap or a hand rinse that would keep skin disinfected for hours and make it easy for all of us to be good. But none has been found. The situation has prompted one expert to propose—only half jokingly—that the best approach may be to give up on hand washing and get people to stop touching patients altogether.

We always hope for the easy fix: the one simple change that will erase a problem in a stroke. But few things in life work this way. Instead, success requires making a hundred small steps go right—one after the other, no slipups, no goofs, everyone pitching in. We are used to thinking of doctoring as a solitary, intellectual task. But making medicine go right is less often like making a difficult diagnosis than like making sure everyone washes their hands.

It is striking to consider how different the history of the operating room after Lister has been from that of the hospital floor after Semmelweis. In the operating room, no one pretends that even 90 percent compliance with scrubbing is good enough. If a single doctor or nurse fails to wash up before coming to the operating table, we are horrified—and certainly not shocked if the patient develops an infection a few days later. Since Lister we have gone even further in our expectations.

We now make sure to use sterile gloves and gowns, masks over our mouths, caps over our hair. We apply antiseptics to the patient's skin and lay down sterile drapes. We put our instruments through steam heat sterilizers or, if any are too delicate to tolerate the autoclave, through chemical sterilizers. We have reinvented almost every detail of the operating room for the sake of antisepsis. We have gone so far as to add an extra person to the team, known as the circulating nurse, whose central job is, essentially, to keep the team antiseptic. Every time an unanticipated instrument is needed for a patient, the team can't stand around waiting for one member to break scrub, pull the thing off a shelf, wash up, and return. So the circulator was invented. Circulators get the extra sponges and instruments, handle the telephone calls, do the paperwork, get help when it's needed. And every time they do, they're not just making the case go more smoothly. They are keeping the patient uninfected. By their very existence, they make sterility a priority in every case.

Stopping the epidemics spreading in our hospitals is not a problem of ignorance—of not having the know-how about what to do. It is a problem of compliance—a failure of an individual to apply that know-how correctly. But achieving compliance is hard. Why, after 140 years, the meticulousness of the operating room has not spread beyond its double doors is a mystery. But the people who are most careful in the surgical theater are frequently the very ones who are least careful on the hospital ward. I know because I have realized I am one of them. I generally try to be as scrupulous about washing my hands when I am outside the operating room as I am inside. And I do pretty well, if I say so myself. But then I blow it. It happens almost every day. I walk into a patient's hospital room, and I'm thinking about what I have to tell him concerning his operation, or about his family, who might be standing there looking worried, or about the funny little joke a resident just told me, and I completely forget about getting a squirt of that gel into my palms, no matter how many laminated reminder signs have been hung on the walls. Sometimes I do remember, but before I can find the dispenser, the patient puts his hand out in greeting and I think it too strange not to go ahead and take it. On occasion I even think, Screw it—I'm late, I have to get a move on, and what difference does it really make what I do this one time?

A few years ago, Paul O'Neill, the former secretary of the Treasury and CEO of the aluminum giant Alcoa, agreed to take over as head of a regional health care initiative in Pittsburgh, Pennsylvania. And he made solving the problem of hospital infections one of his top priorities. To show it could be solved, he arranged for a young industrial engineer named Peter Perreiah to be put on a single forty-bed surgical unit at a Pittsburgh veterans hospital. When he met with the unit's staff, a doctor who worked on the project told me, "Peter didn't ask, 'Why don't you wash your hands?' He asked, 'Why can't you?'" By far the most common answer was time. So, as an engineer, he went about fixing the things that burned up the staff's time. He came up with a just-in-time supply system that kept not only gowns and gloves at the bedside but also gauze and tape and other things the staff needed, so they didn't have to go back and forth out of the room to search for them. Rather than make everyone clean their stethoscopes, notorious carriers of infection, between patients, he arranged for each patient room to have a designated stethoscope on the wall. He helped make dozens of simplifying changes that reduced both the opportunities for spread of infection and the difficulties of staying clean. He made each hospital room work more like an operating room, in other words. He also arranged for a nasal culture to be taken from every patient upon admission, whether the patient seemed infected or not. That way the staff knew which patients carried resistant bacteria and could preemptively use more stringent precautions for them—"search-and-destroy" the strategy is sometimes called. Infection rates for MRSA—the hospital contagion responsible for more deaths than any other—fell almost 90 percent, from four to six infections per month to about that many in an entire year.

Two years later, however, despite encouragement and exhortation, the ideas had spread to only one other unit in the hospital. Those other units didn't have Perreiah. And when he left the original unit for a different project elsewhere, performance on that unit began to slide, too. O'Neill quit the project in frustration. Nothing fundamental had changed.

The belief that something could change did not die, however. Jon Lloyd, a surgeon who had helped Perreiah on the project, continued to puzzle over what to do, and he happened across an article about a Save the Children program to reduce malnutrition in Vietnam. The story seemed to Lloyd to have a lesson for Pittsburgh. The antistarvation program, run by Tufts University nutritionist Jerry Sternin and his wife, Monique, had given up on bringing outside solutions to villages with malnourished children. Over and over, that strategy had failed. Although the know-how to reduce malnutrition was long established—methods to raise more nourishing foods and more effectively feed hungry children—most people proved reluctant to change such fundamental matters as what they fed their children and when just because outsiders said so. The Sternins therefore focused on finding solutions from insiders. They asked small groups of poor villagers to identify who among them had the best-nourished children—who among them had demonstrated what the Sternins termed a "positive deviance" from the norm. The villagers then visited those mothers at home to see exactly what they were doing.

Just that was revolutionary. The villagers discovered that there were well-nourished children among them, despite the poverty, and that those children's mothers were breaking with the locally accepted wisdom in all sorts of ways—feeding their children even when they had diarrhea, for example; giving them several small feedings each day rather than one or two big ones; adding sweet potato greens to the children's rice despite its being considered a low-class food. And the ideas began to spread. They took hold. The program measured the results and posted them in the villages for all to see. In two years, malnutrition dropped 65 to 85 percent in every village the Sternins had been to.

Lloyd was bitten by the positive deviance idea—the idea of building on capabilities people already had rather than telling them how they had to change. By March 2005, he and Perreiah persuaded the veterans hospital leadership in Pittsburgh to try the positive deviance approach with hospital infections. Lloyd even convinced the Sternins to join in. Together they held a series of thirty-minute, small group discussions with health care workers at every level: food service workers, janitors, nurses, doctors, patients themselves. The team began each meeting saying, in essence, "We're here because of the hospital infection problem and we want to know what *you* know about how to solve it." There were no directives, no charts with what the experts thought should be done. "If we had any dogma going in," Jerry Sternin says, "it was: Thou shalt not try to fix anything."

Ideas came pouring out. People told of places where hand-gel dispensers were missing, ways to keep gowns and gloves from running out of supply, nurses who always seemed able to wash their hands and even taught patients to wash their hands, too. Many people said it was the first time anyone had ever asked them what to do. The norms began to shift. When forty new hand-gel dispensers arrived, staff members took charge of putting them up in the right places. Nurses who would never speak up when a doctor failed to wash his or her hands began to do so after learning of other nurses who did. Eight therapists who thought wearing gloves with patients was silly were persuaded by two of their colleagues that it was no big deal. The ideas were not terribly new. "After the eighth group, we began to hear the same things over and over," Sternin says. "But we kept going even if it was group number thirty-three for us, because it was the first time those people had been heard, the first time they had a chance to innovate for themselves."

The team made sure to publicize the ideas and the small victories on the hospital Web site and in newsletters. The team also carried out detailed surveillance—taking nasal cultures from every hospital patient upon admission and upon discharge. They posted the monthly results unit by unit. One year into the experiment—and after years without widespread progress—the entire hospital saw its MRSA wound infection rates drop to zero.

The Robert Wood Johnson Foundation and the Jewish Healthcare Foundation recently launched a multimillion-dollar initiative to implement this approach in ten more hospitals across the country. Lloyd cautions that it remains to be seen whether the Pittsburgh results will last. It also remains to be seen if the success can be duplicated nationally. But nothing else has worked, and this is the most fascinating idea anyone has had to solve the problem in a century.

AT ONE POINT during my tour with Yokoe and Marino, we walked through a regular hospital unit. And I finally began to see the ward the way they do. Flowing in and out of the patients' rooms were physical therapists, patient care assistants, nurses, nutritionists, residents, students. Some were good about washing. Some were not. Yokoe pointed out that three of the eight rooms had bright yellow precaution signs because of patients inside with MRSA or VRE. Only then did I realize we were on the floor of one of my own patients. One of those signs hung on his door.

He was sixty-two years old and had been in the hospital for almost three weeks. He had arrived in shock from another hospital, where an operation had gone awry. I performed an emergency splenectomy for him and then had to go back in again when the bleeding still didn't stop. He had an open abdominal wound and could not eat. He had to receive his nutrition intravenously. He was recovering, though.

Three days after admission, he was out of the intensive care unit. Initial surveillance cultures were completely negative for resistant organisms. New cultures ten days after admission, however, came back positive for both MRSA and VRE. A few days after that, he developed fevers up to 102 degrees. His blood pressure began dropping. His heart rate climbed. He was septic. His central line—his lifeline for nutrition—had become infected, and we had to take it out.

Until that moment, when I stood there looking at the sign on his door, it had not occurred to me that I might have given him that infection. But the truth is I may have. One of us certainly did.

The Mop-Up

P eople underestimate the importance of diligence as a virtue. No doubt this has something to do with how supremely mundane it seems. It is defined as "the constant and earnest effort to accomplish what is undertaken." There is a flavor of simplistic relentlessness to it. And if it were an individual's primary goal in life, that life would indeed seem narrow and unambitious.

Understood, however, as the prerequisite of great accomplishment, diligence stands as one of the most difficult challenges facing any group of people who take on tasks of risk and consequence. It sets a high, seemingly impossible, expectation for performance and human behavior. Yet some in medicine have delivered on that expectation on an almost unimaginable scale. The campaign to eradicate polio in India is just such an instance.

THE INDEX CASE was an eleven-month-old boy with thick black hair his mother liked to comb forward so that the bangs rimmed his round face. His family lives in the southern Indian state of Karnataka, in a village called Upparahalla, along the Tungabhadra River. Dry mountains of teetering rocks can be seen in three directions from the village. It has no running water and little electricity. The boy's mother is illiterate; the father can read only road signs. They are farm laborers, and they live with their three children in a single-room hut of thatch and mud. But the children are well nourished. The mother wears gold and silver earrings. Once in a while, they travel.

In April 2003, the family took a trip north to see relatives. Shortly after they returned, on May 1, the boy developed high fevers and racking bouts of nausea and vomiting. His parents took him to a nearby clinic, where a doctor gave him an antibiotic injection. Two days later, the fevers subsided, but he became unable to move either of his legs. In a panic, the parents took him back to the doctor, who sent him to the district hospital in Bellary, about forty miles away. As the day progressed, the weakness spread through the boy's body. His breathing grew shallow and labored. He lay flat and motionless on his hospital cot.

A doctor at the hospital, following standard procedure in cases of sudden childhood paralysis, phoned a surveillance medical officer with the World Health Organization in Bangalore, the capital of Karnataka. The medical officer made sure that stool specimens were taken and sent for culture to a national laboratory in Mumbai (as Bombay is now called). On June 24, the laboratory results finally came back. A young technical officer with WHO in New Delhi got the call; it was a confirmed case of polio, a disease thought to have been eliminated from southern India, and it set off an alarm.

The World Health Organization is nearly two decades into its campaign to eradicate polio from the world. If the campaign succeeds, it may be mankind's single most ambitious accomplishment. But this is a big if. International organizations are fond of grand-sounding pledges to rid the planet of this or that menace. They nearly always fail, however. The world is too vast and too various to submit to dictates from on high.

Consider the other attempts that have been made to eliminate individual diseases. In 1909, the newly established Rockefeller Foundation launched the first global eradication campaign, an effort to end hookworm disease, using antihelminthic drugs, in fifty-two countries. It didn't work. Today, a billion people—a sixth of the world's population—are infected with hookworm, an intestinal parasite that feeds on human blood. A seventeen-year campaign against yellow fever, led by the Rockefeller Foundation and the United States armed services, had to be abandoned in 1932 when yellow fever was found to have a reservoir outside human beings. (The yellow fever virus persists in mosquitoes' eggs.) In 1955, WHO and UNICEF began a campaign to end yaws, an infectious disease that causes painful, purulent skin ulcers; workers screened 160 million people in sixty-one countries for the disease and treated every case they found with penicillin. A dozen years later, the campaign was dropped when it turned out that silent, subclinical infections were continuing to propagate the disease. Billions of dollars were spent in the fifties and sixties to eradicate malaria; today the disease afflicts more than 300 million people a year.

After a century of effort, the only successful attempt at eradication of a global disease has been the battle against smallpox—a mammoth undertaking that was, just the same, decidedly simpler than the campaign against polio. Smallpox, with its distinctive blisters and vesicles, could be readily and quickly identified; the moment a case appeared, a team could be dispatched to immunize everyone the victim might have come into contact with. That strategy, known as "ring immunization," eradicated the disease by 1979. Polio infections are far harder to identify. For every person who is paralyzed, between two hundred and a thousand infected people come down with little more than a stomach flu—and they remain silently contagious for several weeks after the symptoms abate. Nor is every case of childhood paralysis polio, and it usually takes weeks for stool specimens to be obtained, delivered to a laboratory, and properly tested for the disease. By the time one case has been identified, scores more people have been infected. As a result, the area targeted for polio immunization must be far larger than that for smallpox. And whereas people needed to be vaccinated against smallpox only once for immediate protection, a single dose of polio vaccine does not always take—children with diarrheal illnesses tend to pass the oral vaccine straight through. So a repeat round of immunization is required within four to six weeks. In logistical terms, it's the difference between extinguishing a candle flame and putting out a forest fire.

Despite the obstacles, however, the campaign against polio has made immense progress. Routine vaccination had made polio uncommon in the West, but cases continued to occur in the United States, Canada, and Europe into the 1980s, and the disease remained endemic in large portions of the world. In 1988, more than 350,000 people developed paralytic polio, and at least 70 million were infected with the virus. By 2001, only 498 cases were identified. The whole of the Americas, Europe, and the western Pacific, along with nearly all of Africa and Asia, are currently free of the disease.

In each year since 2001, however, just as the disease was on the verge of being wiped out, an outbreak has flared in some country in Asia or Africa, spilled across borders, and threatened to bring polio roaring back. In 2002, India was that country. Outbreaks in the north produced sixteen hundred polio cases. Four-fifths of all the world's cases occurred there that year. Nonetheless, the belief was that the disease had been isolated to a handful of northern states. Then, in 2003, a boy in south India developed polio—the first case in the state of Karnataka in almost three years. If the disease expanded from there, the campaign would be all but over.

ON JUNE 25, less than twenty-four hours after the report of the Karnataka polio case came in, Sunil Bahl, a WHO physician and technical officer in the Delhi office, sent an e-mail to key people at WHO, at UNICEF, and in the Indian government. It was his job to provide the initial assessment of the facts on the ground. "The case is in an area that has a history of being the worst in Karnataka," he wrote; it had poor routines of immunization and the most polio cases in the early years of the campaign. "Risk of establishment of virus in the area high, unless quick wide and strong measures in the form of a wide mop-up are taken." A "mop-up" is WHO lingo for a targeted campaign to immunize all susceptible children surrounding a new case. It's what is done in an area that has been rendered polio-free through routine immunization but is facing a new infection that threatens to bring the disease back. The campaigns are carried out rapidly, in just three days, to ensure that the vaccine saturates a population and to make it easier to recruit volunteers.

Sunil Bahl sent around a map of the proposed area for the mop-up operation. It covered fifty thousand square miles. Working around the summer holidays and festivals, government officials selected July 27 for the start of the first immunization round. The second round would follow a month later. Brian Wheeler, a thirty-five-year-old Texan who was the chief operations officer for WHO's polio program in India, explained the logistics to me. The Indian government would have to recruit and organize teams of medical workers and volunteers, he said. They would have to be trained in how to administer the vaccine and provided with transportation, vaccine, and insulated coolers and ice packs to keep the vaccine cold. And they would have to fan out and vaccinate every child under five years of age. Anything less than 90 percent coverage of the target population—the percentage needed to shut down transmission—would be considered a failure.

I asked him how many people that would involve.

He checked his budget sheet. The plan, he said, was to employ thirty-seven thousand vaccinators and four thousand health care supervisors, rent two thousand vehicles, supply more than eighteen thousand insulated vaccine carriers, and have the workers go door to door to vaccinate 4.2 million children. In three days.

POLIO IS A disease that strikes children almost exclusively—more than 80 percent of paralysis cases occur in children under age five. It is caused by an intestinal virus; the virus must be ingested to bring about an infection. Once inside the gut, it passes through the lining and takes up residence in nearby lymph nodes. There it multiplies, produces fevers and stomach upset, and passes back into the feces. Those infected can contaminate their clothing, bathing sites, and supplies of drinking water and thereby spread the disease. (The virus can survive as long as sixty days outside the body.)

Poliovirus infects only a few kinds of nerve cells, but what it infects it destroys. In the most dreaded cases, the virus spreads from the bloodstream into the neurons of the brain stem, the cells that allow you to breathe and swallow. To stay alive, a person has to be fed through a tube and ventilated by machine. The nerve cells most commonly attacked, though, are the anterior horn cells of the spinal cord, which control the arms, the legs, and the abdominal muscles. Often, so

many neurons are destroyed that muscle function is eliminated altogether. Tendon reflexes disappear. Limbs hang limp
and useless.

The first effective vaccine for polio was introduced in 1955,
after the largest clinical trial in history. (Jonas Salk's vaccine,
made from killed poliovirus, was given to 440,000 children;
210,000 received a placebo injection, and more than a million
served as unvaccinated controls.) Five years later, Albert Sabin
published the results of an alternative polio vaccine he had
used in an immunization campaign in Toluca, Mexico, a city of
a hundred thousand people, where a polio outbreak was in
progress. His was an oral vaccine, easier to administer than
Salk's injected one. It was also a live vaccine, containing weakened but intact poliovirus, and so it could produce not only
immunity but also a mild contagious infection that would
spread the immunity to others. In just four days, Sabin's team
managed to vaccinate more than 80 percent of the children
under the age of eleven—26,000 children in all. It was a
blitzkrieg assault. Within weeks, polio had disappeared from
the city.

This approach, Sabin argued, could be used to eliminate
polio from entire countries, even the world. The only leader in
the West who took him up on the idea was Fidel Castro. In
1962, Castro's Committee for the Defense of the Revolution
organized 82,366 local committees to carry out a succession of
weeklong house-to-house national immunization campaigns
using the Sabin vaccine. In 1963, only one case of polio occurred in Cuba.

Despite those results, Sabin's grand idea did not catch on
until 1985, when the Pan American Health Organization

launched an initiative to eradicate polio from the Americas. (Six years later, Luis Fermin Tenorio, a two-year-old boy in the town of Pichinaki, Peru, became the last polio victim in the Americas.) In 1988, spurred by the campaign's growing success, WHO committed itself to eradicating polio from the world. That year, Rotary International pledged a quarter of a billion dollars for the effort. (It has since provided 350 million dollars more.) UNICEF agreed to organize the worldwide production and distribution of vaccine. And the United States made the campaign one of the CDC's core initiatives, supplying both expertise and considerable additional funding.

The centerpiece of the effort has been what are called national immunization days—three-day periods when all children under five in a country are immunized, regardless of whether they have received immunization before. In one week in 1997, 250 million children were vaccinated simultaneously in China, India, Bhutan, Pakistan, Bangladesh, Thailand, Vietnam, and Burma. National immunization days have reached as many as half a billion children at one time—almost a tenth of the world's population. Through such efforts—and a reliable network of monitors to detect outbreaks—the WHO campaign has brought the incidence of polio in the world to less than 1 percent of what it used to be.

The striking thing is that WHO doesn't really have the authority to do any of this. It can't tell governments what to do. It hires no vaccinators, distributes no vaccine. It is a small Geneva bureaucracy run by several hundred international delegates whose annual votes tell the organization what to do but not how to do it. In India, a nation of a billion people, WHO employs 250 physicians around the country to work on polio monitoring. The only substantial resource that WHO has cultivated is information and expertise. I didn't understand how this could suffice. Then I went to Karnataka.

FOR THE THREE days of the mop-up, I traveled through Karnataka with Pankaj Bhatnagar, a WHO pediatrician whose job was to see that the operation was properly executed. He is in his forties, with a slight paunch and an easy, genial manner. The work can be a tricky business, he explained as we waited in Delhi for our flight south. WHO distributes much of the money for mop-up operations. UNICEF provides the vaccines. Rotary of India prints the banners and advocates locally for the cause. But the operation itself is run by people none of these organizations control: government health officials who must hire the thousands of vaccinators, train them properly, and send them from house to house.

We took a plane to Bangalore, then traveled eight hours overnight by train to Bellary, a crowded, dusty town that is the district seat for Upparahalla. At a small, strange hotel there (it had a safari theme), Pankaj convened the members of his team over breakfast. To monitor the immunization of four million children, he had just four people: three young medical officers and himself. They were the only ones available who spoke Kanada, the local language. The medical officers finished their breakfast of idli and dosa and lit up cigarettes (in India, it seems, half the doctors who work in public health smoke), and then Pankaj asked for a status report.

Since the index case was identified, he was told, four more cases of confirmed polio had appeared in the region, including another child in Upparahalla, and four "hot" cases were awaiting confirmatory testing. Of the thirteen districts targeted for mop-ups, Bellary accounted for all but one of the cases.

"Then we must concentrate our monitoring in this district," Pankaj said. "This is now the place with the most intense transmission of polio in the world." Another doctor pulled out some figures on the area. Bellary district, he told Pankaj, has a population of 2,965,459, with 542 villages and nine urban towns. Fifty-two percent of the males and 74 percent of the females are illiterate. There are just ninety-nine doctors in the district public health system. He turned to a map. The polio cases, he said, were clustered in a triangle of villages around Siriguppa, a small, slum-ridden town about forty miles away.

Pankaj made his assignments. For the mop-up, he would check on progress in at least Upparahalla, a village called Sirigere where polio had appeared, the two urban areas with hot cases, and a mine in Chitradurga, where vaccinators might have particular difficulties gaining entry because the housing was on the property of a private company. He assigned the remaining villages to the others and asked them to follow up behind him for a second check in Upparahalla and the urban areas. The group then split up. By eight thirty in the morning, Pankaj and I were on the road.

WE HAD A rented four-wheel-drive Toyota and a betel-nut-chewing driver who waited until we were an hour down a pitted road to tell us that the battery was dead. Whenever the engine was turned off, he said, we'd need to push-start the car. Pankaj thought this was funny.

The terrain outside the windows was baked by the hot sun, and the hills were desert-lizard brown. The monsoon had failed to come this year. Only the few fields that had drip irrigation looked green. It took us about two hours to travel the thirty-five miles to Sirigere, a village of mud-walled huts jammed up against one another. There was garbage in the alleyways, and dust-faced children were playing everywhere. Pankaj had the driver stop at a group of dwellings seemingly at random. Marked in chalk on each door was a number, a "P," and that day's date. The number was the house number. The "P" meant that the vaccinators had come, identified all the children under the age of five who lived in the house, and vaccinated them—that very day, according to the date marked. Pankaj took out a pad of paper and strode over to one of the huts. He asked the young woman at the door how many children lived there. One, she said. He asked to see the child. When she found him, Pankaj took his hand and noted the black ink mark on the nail bed of his little finger—it's how the vaccinators tag the children who have received polio drops. Was any other child in the fields? Away at a relative's? No, she said. He asked if her boy had received routine immunizations before today. No, she said. Had she heard about the polio case in town? She had. Had she heard about the vaccination team before the workers arrived at the door? She had not. He thanked her and wrote all the information down on a form before moving on.

Several houses later, Pankaj said that, so far, the workers

had done their job. But he was disturbed that no one knew the vaccinators were coming that day. In addition to putting up banners (we'd seen a couple hanging as we came into the village), workers were supposed to use "miking" to reach the illiterate—auto-rickshaws with loudspeakers playing tapes announcing the upcoming campaign. Without that warning, some people would turn away the vaccinators knocking on their doors.

Going around to a few more huts, we bumped into a vaccination team—a social welfare worker wearing sandals, a blue sari, and a flower in her hair, and a younger, college-student volunteer with a flower in her hair, too, and a square blue cold box of vaccine slung over her shoulder. They were standing in front of a hut they'd marked with an "X" instead of a "P"—the woman of the house had said that three children lived there, but one was absent and could not be vaccinated. Pankaj asked the vaccinators to open their cold box. He checked the freezer packs inside—still frozen, despite the heat. He inspected the individual vaccine vials—still fresh. There was a gray-and-white target sign on each vial. Did they know what it meant? That the vaccine was still good, they said. What does it look like when the vaccine expires? The white inside the target turns gray or black, they said. Right answer. Pankaj moved on.

We went to the home of the village's recent polio case. The girl was eighteen months old and silent. The mother, pregnant and with a three-year-old boy clinging to her side, laid her down on her back so that we could examine her. Neither leg would move. Lifting each one, I felt no resistance in the child's hips, her knees, her ankles. Only four weeks had passed since she was stricken. She almost certainly was still contagious.

Pankaj found three children visiting the house. He checked each of their hands. None had received polio drops yet.

WE GAVE THE four-wheel drive a push and made our way to Sirigere's primary health center, a few miles outside the village. It was a drab, unpainted, three-room concrete building. The center's medical officer met us at the door. About forty years old, with ironed slacks, a buttoned short-sleeve shirt, and the only college education in the area, he seemed eager to have our company. He offered tea and tried to make small talk. But Pankaj was all business. "May I see your microplan?" he asked before we had even sat down. He was referring to the block-by-block plan drawn up by each local officer. It is the key to how the operation is organized.

The medical officer's microplan was a sheaf of ragged paper, with marker-drawn maps and penciled-in tables. The first page said that he had recruited twenty-two teams of two vaccinators each to cover a population of 34,144 people. "How do you know this population estimate is right?" Pankaj asked. The officer replied that he'd done a house-to-house survey. Pankaj looked at the map—the villages in the area were spread out over more than ten miles. "How do you distribute the vaccine to the vaccinators who are far away?" By vehicle, the officer said. "How many vehicles do you have?" Two, he said. "What are the vehicles?" One was an ambulance. The other was a rented car. "And how does the supervisor get out to the field?" There was a pause. The officer shuffled through the microplan. More silence. He did not know.

Pankaj went on. Twenty-two teams would require about a hundred ice packs per day, or three hundred ice packs altogether. "Why did you budget for only a hundred and fifty ice packs?" We are freezing them overnight for the next day, the officer explained. "Where?" He showed Pankaj his deep freezer. Pankaj opened it up and pulled out the thermometer, which revealed that the temperature was above freezing. The electricity goes out, the officer explained. "What is your plan for that?" He had a generator. But when pressed to show it he was forced to admit that it wasn't really working, either.

Pankaj is not a physically imposing man. He has a boyish mop of thick black hair, parted almost down the center, and sometimes it sticks up. He has programed his cell phone to play the James Bond theme when it rings. When we're driving, he points out the monkeys we pass. He makes jokes. He laughs with his head tilted back. But in the field his demeanor is grave and taciturn. He doesn't tell people if their answers are good or bad. He keeps everyone on edge. I had an impulse to tell the medical officer that he was doing okay. But Pankaj seemed to make a point of saying nothing to fill the silences.

In Siriguppa, where two of the hot cases had appeared, we walked the neighborhoods with another medical officer. Siriguppa is a dense, urbanized town of windowless concrete-block tenements, rusting corrugated-metal lean-tos, and some forty-three thousand people. We had to fight our way through narrow streets crowded with water buffalo, motorcycles, braying goats, and fruit sellers. There was electricity here, I noticed, running through wires that drooped from scattered utility poles, and the sound of televisions poured out from some of the houses.

The two hot cases, we found, were in a small Muslim enclave that had sprouted up a few months earlier. Going door to door, Pankaj learned that almost none of the enclave's children had received routine immunizations. Some of the families seemed suspicious of us, answering questions tersely or trying to avoid us altogether. We found one boy whom the vaccinators had missed. Pankaj was concerned other children might have been hidden. The previous year, rumors had circulated among Muslims that the Indian government was giving different drops to their male children in order to make them infertile. The rumors were thought to have been quashed by an education campaign and greater Muslim involvement in the immunization program. But one had to wonder.

Later, walking with a local doctor and a vaccination team through a village called Balkundi, we came to the home of a small, pretty woman who had rings on her toes and a baby held loosely on her hip. Another child, a boy of about three, stood nearby, staring at our little crowd. Neither child had been vaccinated, so Pankaj asked if we could give them the polio drops. No, she said. She did not appear angry or afraid. Pankaj asked if she knew that a case of polio had appeared in her neighborhood. Yes, she said. But she still didn't want the drops given. Why? She would not say. Pankaj said OK, thanked her for her time, and moved on to the next house.

"That's it?" I asked.

"Yes," he said.

The local doctor had stayed behind, however, and when

we looked back he was shouting at the mother: "Are you stupid? Your children will become paralyzed. They will die."

It was the one time I saw Pankaj angry. He walked back and confronted the doctor. "Why are you shouting?" Pankaj demanded. "Before, she was listening, at least. But now? She's not going to listen anymore."

"She is illiterate!" the doctor shot back, embarrassed to be rebuked so openly. "She doesn't know what is right for her child!"

"What does that matter?" Pankaj replied. "Your shouting doesn't help anything. And neither will a story going around that we are forcing drops on people."

So far, few were refusing the drops, and that was good enough, he told me later. A single nasty rumor could destroy the whole operation.

ONE DIFFICULT QUESTION came up repeatedly—from local doctors, from villagers, from workers trudging house to house. The question was: Why? Why this huge polio campaign when what we need is—fill in the blank here—clean water (diarrheal illness kills 500,000 Indian children per year), better nutrition (half of children under three have stunted growth), working septic systems (which would help prevent polio as well as other diseases), irrigation (so a single rainless season would not impoverish farming families)? We saw neighborhoods that had had outbreaks of malaria, tuberculosis, cholera. But no one important had come to visit in years. Now one case of polio occurs and the infantry marches in?

There are some stock answers. We can do it all, goes one.

We can eradicate polio and do better on the other fronts. In reality, though, choices are made. For that whole week, for instance, doctors in northern Karnataka had all but shut down their primary health clinics in order to carry out the polio vaccination work.

Pankaj relies on a somewhat more persuasive line of argument: that ending polio is in itself worthwhile. In one village, I watched a resident demand to know why the government and WHO weren't combating malnutrition there instead. There was only so much they could do, Pankaj said. "And if you're starving, becoming paralyzed certainly isn't going to help."

Still, you could make the same claim for almost any human problem that you decide to tackle—blindness or cancer or, for that matter, kidney stones. ("If you're starving, kidney pain certainly isn't going to help.") And then there is the issue of money. So far the campaign has cost three billion dollars worldwide, more than six hundred dollars a case. To put that in perspective, the Indian government's total budget for health care in 2003 came to four dollars per person. Stopping the very last case of polio, one official told me, might cost as much as two hundred million dollars. Even if the campaign succeeds in the eradication of polio, it is entirely possible that more lives would be saved in the future if the money were spent on, say, building proper sewage systems or improving basic health services.

What's more, success is by no means assured. WHO has had to extend its target date for eradication from 2000 to 2002 to 2005 and now is having to extend it again. In these last years of the campaign, more and more money has been spent chasing the few hundred cases that keep popping up. A certain weariness is bound to settle in. Around twenty-four million children are born in India each year, creating a new pool of potential polio victims the size of Venezuela's entire population. Just to stay caught up, a mammoth campaign to immunize every child under the age of five has to be planned each year. The truth is, no cost-benefit calculus can assure us just now that the money is well spent.

Yet for all these reservations, the campaign has averted an estimated five million cases of paralytic polio thus far—a momentous achievement in itself. And although erasing the disease from the world is a grand, perhaps even absurd ambition, it remains a feasible task and one of the few things we as a civilization can do that would benefit mankind forever. The eradication of smallpox will last as an enduring gift to all who are to come, and now, perhaps, the eradication of polio can, too.

But this means we must actually get down to that final polio case. Otherwise, the efforts of the hundreds of thousands of volunteers, and the billions spent will have amounted to nothing—or maybe worse than nothing. To fail at this venture would put into question the very ideal of eradication.

Beneath the ideal is the gruelingly unglamorous and uncertain work. If the eradication of polio is our monument, it is a monument to the perfection of performance—to showing what can be achieved by diligent attention to detail coupled with great ambition. There is a system, and it has eradicated polio in countries with far worse conditions than I was seeing in India—for example, in Bangladesh, in Vietnam, in Rwanda, in Zimbabwe. Polio was eradicated from Angola in the midst of a civil war. An outbreak in Kandahar in 2002 was halted by a WHO-led mop-up operation despite the Afghan war. In 2006, new mop-ups took place in northern Nigeria, where polio remains endemic and periodically spills into neighboring countries. In India, Pankaj told me, there have been campaigns on camels in the Thar Desert of Rajasthan, in jeeps among the tribal communities of the Jharkhand forests, on power boats through flooded regions of Assam and Meghalaya, on Navy cruisers traveling to remote islands in the Bay of Bengal. During our own mop-up, we covered about a thousand miles in the three days of going town to town. Pankaj worked his mobile phone almost constantly. Armed with the information he provided, state officials arranged deliveries from ice factories to teams at risk of running short of ice packs and extended the mop-up by an additional day in one area where the local officer had severely underestimated the population to be vaccinated. Four miles outside the village of Balkundi, we came upon a cluster of makeshift shanties for migrant laborers, not seen on any maps. When we checked the children, though, they all had the vaccinators' ink marks on their pinkies. At Chitradurga, we found the mines in decay, but state officials had made sure that the company gave the vaccinators access to the workers' compound. With some searching, we discovered a few children here and there. Every one of them had received the vaccine, too.

By the end of the mop-up, UNICEF officials had distributed more than five million doses of fresh vaccine through the thirteen districts. Television, radio, and local newspapers had been blanketed with public service announcements. Rotary of India had printed and delivered 25,000 banners, 6,000 posters, and more than 650,000 handbills. And 4 million of the targeted 4.2 million children had been successfully vaccinated.

In 2005, India had just sixty-six new cases of polio. Pankaj and his colleagues believe that they're finally closing in on their goal of eradication in India. And as India goes, so might the world.

STILL, THERE IS no denying the dimensions of what Pankaj and his colleagues are up against. Pankaj says that he has seen more than a thousand cases of polio in his career as a pediatrician. When we drove through the villages and towns, he could pick out polio victims at a glance. They were everywhere, I began to realize: the beggar with two emaciated legs folded under him, rolling by on a wooden cart; the man dragging his leg like a club down the street; the passerby with a contracted arm tucked against his side.

On the second day of the mop-up, we reached Upparahalla, the village where the Karnataka outbreak had started. The first, index case of polio was now a fourteen-month-old boy with a healthy, almost muscular thickness about his upper body; after the first few days of his infection, his breathing had returned to normal. But when his mother put him down on his stomach you could see that his legs were withered. With the exercises the nurses had taught her to do with him, he had regained enough movement in his left leg to be able to crawl, but his right leg dragged limply behind him.

Making our way around the open sewage in Upparahalla, the mud-covered pigs, the cows resting curled up like cats with their heads on their hooves, we found the neighbor girl who had come down with polio after the boy. She was eighteen months old, with a big, worried face, perfect white teeth, and short, spiky hair. She was wearing small gold earrings and a yellow-and-brown checked dress. She squirmed in her mother's arms, but her legs only dangled beneath her dress. Her mother wore an impassive expression as she stood before us in the sun, holding her paralyzed child. Pankaj gently asked her if the girl had ever received polio drops—perhaps she'd got the vaccine but it had not taken. The mother said that a health worker had come around with polio drops a few weeks before her daughter became sick. But she had heard from other villagers that children were getting fevers from the drops. So she refused the vaccination. A look of profound sadness now swept over her. She had not understood, she said, staring down at the ground.

Eventually, Pankaj continued onward, checking on the vaccinators going door to door. Then, when he was finished, we left. The road heading out of the village was a red dirt track and we rattled over it with our wheels in the ruts that the bullock carts had made.

"What will you do when polio is finally gone?" I asked Pankaj.

"Well, there is always measles," he said.

Casualties of War

Each Tuesday, the U.S. Department of Defense provides an online update of American military casualties from the wars in Iraq and Afghanistan. According to this update, as of December 8, 2006, a total of 26,547 service members had suffered battle injuries. Of these, 2,662 died; 10,839 lived but could not return to duty; and 13,085 were less severely wounded and returned to duty within seventy-two hours. These figures represent, by a considerable margin, the largest burden of casualties our military medical personnel have had to cope with since the Vietnam War.

When U.S. combat deaths in Iraq reached the two-thousand mark in September 2005, the event captured worldwide attention. Combat deaths are seen as a measure of the magnitude and dangerousness of war, just as murder rates are seen as a measure of the magnitude and dangerousness of violence in our communities. Both, however, are weak proxies. Little recognized is how fundamentally important the medical system is—and not just the enemy's weaponry—in determining whether or not someone dies. U.S. homicide rates, for example, have dropped in recent years to levels unseen since the mid-1960s. Yet aggravated assaults, particularly with firearms, have more than tripled during that period. A key mitigating factor appears to be the trauma care provided: more people may be getting shot, but doctors are saving even more of them. Mortality from gun assaults has fallen from 16 percent in 1964 to 5 percent today.

We have seen a similar evolution in war. Though firepower has increased, lethality has decreased. In the Revolutionary War, American soldiers faced bayonets and single-shot rifles, and 42 percent of the battle wounded died. In World War II, American soldiers were hit with grenades, bombs, shells, and machine guns, yet only 30 percent of the wounded died. By the Korean War, the weaponry was certainly no less terrible, but the mortality rate for combat-injured soldiers fell to 25 percent.

Over the next half century, we saw little further progress. Through the Vietnam War (with its 153,303 combat wounded and 47,424 combat dead) and even the 1990–91 Persian Gulf War (with its 467 wounded and 147 dead), mortality rates for the battle injured remained at 24 percent. Our technology to save the wounded seemed to have barely kept up with the technology inflicting the wounds.

The military wanted desperately to find ways to do better. The most promising approach was to focus on discovering new treatments and technologies. In the previous century, that was where progress had been found—in the discovery of new anesthetic agents and vascular surgery techniques for World War I soldiers, in the development of better burn treatments, blood transfusion methods, and penicillin for World War II soldiers, in the availability of a broad range of antibiotics for Korean War soldiers. The United States accordingly invested hundreds of millions of dollars in numerous new possibilities: the development of blood substitutes and freeze-dried plasma (for infusion when fresh blood is not available), gene therapies for traumatic wounds, medications to halt lung injury, miniaturized systems to monitor and transmit the vital signs of soldiers in the field.

Few if any of these have yet come to fruition, however, and none were responsible for what we have seen in the current wars in Iraq and Afghanistan: a marked, indeed historic, reduction in the lethality of battle wounds. Although more U.S. soldiers have been wounded in combat in the current war than in the Revolutionary War, the War of 1812, and the Spanish-American War combined, and more than in the first four years of military involvement in Vietnam, we have had substantially fewer deaths. Just 10 percent of wounded American soldiers have died.

How military medical teams have achieved this is important to think about. They have done it despite having no fundamentally new technologies or treatments since the Persian Gulf War. And they have done it despite difficulties with the supply of medical personnel. For its entire worldwide mission, the army had only about 120 general surgeons available on active duty and two hundred in the reserves in 2005. To support the 130,000 to 150,000 troops fighting in Iraq, it has been able to put no more than thirty to fifty general surgeons and ten to fifteen orthopedic surgeons on the ground. And these surgeons and their teams have been up against devastating injuries.

I got a sense of the extent of the injuries during a visit to Walter Reed Army Medical Center in Washington, D.C., in the fall of 2004, when I was invited to sit in on what the doctors call their "War Rounds." Every Thursday, the Walter Reed surgeons hold a telephone conference with army surgeons in Baghdad to review the American casualties received in Washington. The case list for discussion the day I visited included one gunshot wound, one antitank-mine injury, one grenade injury, three rocket-propelled-grenade injuries, four mortar injuries, eight improvised explosive device (IED) injuries, and seven with no cause of injury noted. None of these soldiers was more than twenty-five years of age. The least seriously wounded was a nineteen-year-old who had sustained extensive blast and penetrating injuries to his face and neck from a mine. Other cases included a soldier with a partial hand amputation; one with a massive blast injury that amputated his right leg at the hip, a through-knee amputation of his left leg, and an open pelvic wound; one with bullet wounds to his left kidney and colon; one with bullet wounds under his arm requiring axillary artery and vein reconstruction; and one with a shattered spleen, a degloving scalp laceration, and a through-and-through tongue laceration. These are terrible and formidable injuries. Nonetheless, all were saved.

★   ★   ★

IF THE ANSWER to how was not to be found in new technologies, it did not seem to reside in any special skills of military doctors, either. George Peoples is a forty-two-year-old surgical oncologist who was my chief resident when I was a surgical intern. In October 2001, after the September 11 attacks on the World Trade Center and the Pentagon, he led the first surgical team into Afghanistan. He returned after service there only to be sent to Iraq, in March 2003, with ground forces invading from Kuwait through the desert to Baghdad. He had gone to the U.S. Military Academy at West Point for college, Johns Hopkins Medical School in Baltimore, Brigham and Women's Hospital in Boston for surgical residency, and then M. D. Anderson Cancer Center in Houston for a cancer surgery fellowship. He owed the army eighteen years of service when he finally finished his training, and neither I nor anyone I know ever heard him bemoan that commitment. In 1998, he was assigned to Walter Reed, where he soon became chief of surgical oncology. Peoples was known in training for three things: his unflappability, his intellect (he had published seventeen papers on work toward a breast cancer vaccine before he finished his training), and the five children he and his wife had during his residency. He was not known, however, for any particular expertise in trauma surgery. Before being deployed, he hadn't seen a gunshot wound since residency, and even then, he never saw anything like the injuries he saw in Iraq. His practice at Walter Reed centered on breast surgery. Yet in Iraq, he and his team managed to save historic numbers of wounded.

"How is this possible?" I asked him. I asked his colleagues, too. I asked everyone I met who had worked on medical teams in the war. And what they described revealed an intriguing effort to do something we in civilian medicine do spottily at best: to make a science of performance, to investigate and improve how well they use the knowledge and technologies they already have at hand. The doctors told me of simple, almost banal changes that produced enormous improvements.

One such change involved Kevlar vests, for example. There is nothing new about Kevlar. It has been around since the late 1970s. Urban police forces began using Kevlar vests in the early 1980s. American troops had them during the Persian Gulf War. A sixteen-pound Kevlar flak vest will protect a person's "body core"—the heart, the lungs, the abdominal organs—from blasts, blunt force trauma, and penetrating injuries. But researchers examining wound registries from the Persian Gulf War found that wounded soldiers had been coming in to medical facilities without their Kevlar on. *They hadn't been wearing their vests.* So orders were handed down holding commanders responsible for ensuring that their soldiers always wore the vests—however much they might complain about how hot or heavy or uncomfortable the vests were. Once the soldiers began wearing them more consistently, the percentage killed on the battlefield dropped instantly.

A second, key discovery came in much the same way, by looking more carefully at how the system was performing. Colonel Ronald Bellamy, a surgeon with the army's Borden Institute, examined the statistics of the Vietnam War and found that helicopter evacuation had reduced the transport time for injured soldiers to hospital care from an average of over eleven hours in World War II to under an hour. And once they got to surgical care, only 3 percent died. Yet 24 percent of wounded soldiers died in all, and that was because transport time to surgical care under an hour still wasn't fast enough. Civilian surgeons talk of having a "Golden Hour" during which most trauma victims can be saved if treatment is started. But battlefield injuries are so much more severe—the blood loss in particular—that wounded soldiers have only a "Golden Five Minutes," Bellamy reported. Vests could extend those five minutes. But the recent emphasis on leaner, faster-moving military units moving much farther ahead of supply lines and medical facilities was only going to make evacuation to medical care more difficult and time-consuming. Outcomes for the wounded were in danger of getting worse rather than better.

The army therefore turned to an approach that had been used in isolated instances going back as far as World War II: something called Forward Surgical Teams (FSTs). These are small teams, consisting of just twenty people: three general surgeons, one orthopedic surgeon, two nurse anesthetists, three nurses, plus medics and other support personnel. In Iraq and Afghanistan, they travel in six Humvees directly behind the troops, right out onto the battlefield. They carry three lightweight, Deployable Rapid-Assembly Shelter ("drash") tents that attach to one another to form a nine-hundred-square-foot hospital facility. Supplies to immediately resuscitate and operate on the wounded are in five black nylon backpacks: an ICU pack, a surgical-technician pack, an anesthesia pack, a general-surgery pack, and an orthopedic pack. They hold sterile instruments, anesthesia equipment, medicines, drapes, gowns, catheters, and a handheld unit that allows clinicians to measure a complete blood count, electrolytes, or blood gases with a drop of blood. FSTs also carry a small ultrasound machine, portable monitors, transport ventilators, an oxygen concentrator providing up to 50 percent pure oxygen, twenty units of packed red blood cells for transfusion, and six roll-up stretchers with litter stands. All of this is ordinary medical equipment. The teams must forgo many technologies normally available to a surgeon, such as angiography and radiography equipment. (Orthopedic surgeons, for example, have to detect fractures by feel.) But they can go from rolling to having a fully functioning hospital with two operating tables and four ventilator-equipped recovery beds in under sixty minutes.

Peoples led the 274th FST, which traveled 1,100 miles with troops during the invasion of Iraq. The team set up in Nasiriyah, Najaf, Karbala, and points along the way in the southern desert, then in Mosul in the north, and finally in Baghdad. According to its logs, the unit cared for 132 U.S. and 74 Iraqi casualties (22 of the Iraqis were combatants, 52 civilians) over those initial weeks. Some days were quiet, others overwhelming. On one day in Nasiriyah, the team received ten critically wounded soldiers, among them one with right-lower-extremity shrapnel injuries; one with gunshot wounds to the stomach, small bowel, and liver; another with gunshot wounds to the gallbladder, liver, and transverse colon; one with shrapnel in the neck, chest, and back; one with a gunshot wound through the rectum; and two with extremity gunshot wounds. The next day, fifteen more casualties arrived.

Peoples described to me how radically the new system changed the way he and his team took care of the wounded. On the arrival of the wounded, they carried out the standard Advanced Trauma Life Support protocols that all civilian trauma teams follow. However, because of the high proportion of penetrating wounds—80 percent of casualties seen by the 274th FST had gunshot wounds, shrapnel injuries, or blast injuries—lifesaving operative management is required far more frequently than in civilian trauma centers. The FST's limited supplies provided only for a short period of operative care for a soldier and no more than six hours of postoperative intensive care. So the unit's members focused on damage control, not definitive repair. They packed off liver injuries with gauze pads to stop the bleeding, put temporary plastic tubes in bleeding arteries to shunt the blood past the laceration, stapled off perforated bowel, washed out dirty wounds—whatever was necessary to control contamination and stop hemorrhage. They sought to keep their operations under two hours in length. Then, having stabilized the injuries, they shipped the soldier off—often still anesthetized, on a ventilator, the abdominal wound packed with gauze and left open, bowel loops not yet connected, blood vessels still needing repair—to another team at the next level of care.

They had available to them two Combat Support Hospitals (or CSHs—"CaSHes"—as they call them) in four locations for that next level of care. These are 248-bed hospitals typically with six operating tables, some specialty surgery services, and radiology and laboratory facilities. Mobile hospitals as well, they arrive in modular units by air, tractor trailer, or ship and can be fully functional in twenty-four to forty-eight hours. Even at the CSH level, the goal is not necessarily definitive repair. The maximal length of stay is intended to be three days. Wounded American soldiers requiring longer care are transferred to what's called a level IV hospital—one was established in Kuwait and one in Rota, Spain, but the main one is in

Landstuhl, Germany. Those expected to require more than thirty days of treatment are transferred home, mainly to Walter Reed or to Brooke Army Medical Center in San Antonio, Texas. Iraqi prisoners and civilians, however, remain in the CSHs through recovery.

The system took some getting used to. Surgeons at every level initially tended to hold on to their patients, either believing that they could provide definitive care themselves or not trusting that the next level could do so. ("Trust no one" is the mantra we all learn to live by in surgical training.) According to statistics from Walter Reed, during the first few months of the war it took the most severely injured soldiers—those who clearly needed prolonged and extensive care—an average of eight days to go from the battlefield to a U.S. facility. Gradually, however, surgeons embraced the wisdom of the approach. The average time from battlefield to arrival in the United States is now less than four days. (In Vietnam, it was forty-five days.) And the system has worked.

One airman I met during my visit to Washington had experienced a mortar attack outside Balad on September 11, 2004, and ended up on a Walter Reed operating table just thirty-six hours later. In extremis from bilateral thigh injuries, abdominal wounds, shrapnel in the right hand, and facial injuries, he was taken from the field to the nearby 31st CSH in Balad. Bleeding was controlled, resuscitation with intravenous fluids and blood begun, a guillotine amputation at the thigh performed. He received exploratory abdominal surgery and, because a ruptured colon was found, a colostomy. His abdomen was left open, with a clear plastic covering sewn on. A note was taped to him explaining exactly what the surgeons had done. He was then taken to Landstuhl by an air force critical care transport team. When he arrived in Germany, army surgeons determined that he would require more than thirty days of recovery, if he made it at all. Resuscitation was continued, a quick further washout performed, and then he was sent on to Walter Reed. There, after weeks in intensive care and multiple operations to complete the repairs, he survived. This sequence of care is unprecedented, and so is the result. Injuries like his were unsurvivable in previous wars.

But if mortality is low, the human cost remains high. The airman lost one leg above the knee, the other at the hip, his right hand, and part of his face. How he and others like him will be able to live and function remains an open question. His abdominal injuries prevented him from being able to lift himself out of bed or into a wheelchair. With only one hand, he could not manage his colostomy. We have never faced having to rehabilitate people with such extensive wounds. We are only beginning to learn what to do to make a life worth living possible for them.

ON APRIL 4, 2004, after four private military contractors were killed and their bodies mutilated in Fallujah, just to the west of Baghdad, three marine battalions launched an attack to take control of the city from the fifteen to twenty thousand insurgents operating there. Five days later, after intense fighting and protests from Iraqi authorities, the White House ordered the troops to retreat. The marines staged a second attack seven months afterward, on November 9. Four marine battalions and two army mechanized infantry battalions with some twelve thousand troops in all fought street-to-street against snipers and groups of insurgents hiding among the two hundred mosques and fifty thousand buildings of the city. The city was recaptured in about a week, although fighting continued for weeks afterward. During the two battles for Fallujah, American forces suffered more than 1,100 casualties in all, the insurgents a still-untold number. To care for the wounded, fewer than twenty trauma surgeons were in the vicinity; just two neurosurgeons were available in the entire country. Marine and army forward surgical teams received some of the wounded but were quickly overwhelmed. Others were transported by two-hundred-mile-per-hour Blackhawk medevac helicopters directly to combat support hospitals, about half of them to the 31st CSH in Baghdad.

Another of the surgeons I had trained with in Boston, Michael Murphy, was a reservist on duty there at the time. A North Carolina vascular surgeon, he had signed up with the army reserves in June 2004. In October, he got a call from central command. "I left Durham on a Sunday, and a week later I was in a convoy going down the Irish Road in Iraq with an M9 pistol in my hand, wondering what I had gotten myself into," he later told me.

The moment he arrived at the 31st CSH—he still had his bags in his hands—Murphy was sent to the operating room to help with a soldier who had shrapnel injuries to the abdomen, both legs missing, and a spouting arterial injury in one arm. It was the worst injury Murphy had ever seen. The physicians, nurses, and medics took him in like a wet pup. They worked together as more of a team than he'd ever experienced. "In two weeks, I went from a guy who was scared to death about whether I was going to cut it to the point where I was the most comfortable I had ever felt as a surgeon," he says.

With Operation Phantom Fury, as the military called the November battle for Fallujah, the CSH was strained almost to the breaking point. "The wounded came in waves of five, ten, fifteen every two hours," Murphy says. The CSH had twenty-five beds in the ER, five operating tables, and one critical care team, and that did not seem nearly enough. But they made do. Surgeons and emergency physicians saw the worst casualties as they came in. Family physicians, pediatricians, and even ophthalmologists—whoever was available—stabilized the less seriously injured. The surgical teams up in the operating rooms stuck to damage control surgery to keep the soldiers moving off the operating tables. Once stabilized, the American wounded were evacuated to Landstuhl. One-third of the patients were Iraqi wounded, and they had to stay until beds in Iraqi hospitals were found, if they were civilians or security forces, or until they were recovered enough to go to prison facilities, if they were insurgents. In the thick of it, Murphy says, he and his colleagues worked for forty-eight hours with little more than half-hour breaks here and there, grabbed some sleep, then worked for forty-eight hours more.

Six hundred and nine American soldiers were wounded in the first six days of the November battle. Nonetheless, the military teams managed to keep the overall death rate at just 10 percent. Of 1,100 American soldiers wounded during the twin battles for Fallujah, the teams saved all but 104—a stunning accomplishment. And it was only possible through a kind of resolute diligence that is difficult to imagine. Think, for example, about the fact that we even know the statistics of what happened to the wounded in Fallujah. It is only because the medical teams took the time, despite the chaos and their fatigue, to fill out their logs describing the injuries and their outcomes. At the 31st CSH, three senior physicians took charge of collecting the data; they input more than seventy-five different pieces of information on every casualty—all so they could later analyze the patterns in what had happened to the soldiers and how effective the treatments had been. "We had a little doctors' room with two computers," Murphy recalls. "I remember I'd see those guys late at night, sometimes in the early hours of the morning, putting the data in."

We do little tracking like this here at home. Ask a typical American hospital what its death and complications rates for surgery were during the last six months and it cannot tell you. Few institutions ask their doctors to collect this information. Doctors don't have time, I am tempted to say. But then I remember those surgeons in Baghdad in the dark hours at their PCs. Knowing their results was so important to them that they skipped sleep to gather the data. They understood that such vigilance over the details of their own performance—the same kind of vigilance practiced by WHO physicians working to eradicate polio from the world and the Pittsburgh VA hospital units seeking to eliminate hospital infections—offered the only chance to do better.

As THE WAR continued, medical teams were forced to confront numerous unanticipated circumstances. The war went on far longer than planned, the volume of wounded soldiers increased, and the nature of the injuries changed. The data,

however, proved to be of crucial importance. Surgeons following the trauma logs began to see, for example, a dismayingly
high incidence of blinding injuries. Soldiers had been directed
to wear eye protection, but they evidently found the issued
goggles too ugly. As one soldier put it, "They look like something a Florida senior citizen would wear." So the military
bowed to fashion and switched to cooler-looking Wiley-brand
ballistic eyewear. The rate of eye injuries decreased markedly.

Military doctors also found that blast injuries from suicide bombs, land mines, and other IEDs were increasing and
were proving particularly difficult to manage. IEDs often produce a combination of penetrating, blunt, and burn injuries.
The shrapnel include not only nails, bolts, and the like but also
dirt, clothing, even bone from assailants. Victims of IED attacks can exsanguinate from multiple seemingly small wounds.
The military therefore updated first aid kits to include emergency bandages that go on like a tourniquet over a wound and
can be cinched down with one hand by the soldiers themselves. A newer bandage impregnated with a material that can
clot blood more quickly was distributed. The surgical teams
that receive blast injury victims learned to pack all the bleeding sites with gauze before starting abdominal surgery or
other interventions. And they began to routinely perform se-
rial operative washouts of wounds to ensure adequate removal of infectious debris.

This is not to say military physicians always found solutions. The logs have revealed many problems for which they
do not yet have good answers. Early in the war in Iraq, for example, Kevlar vests proved dramatically effective in preventing
torso injuries. Surgeons, however, found that IEDs were caus-

ing blast injuries that extended upward under the armor and inward through underarm vents. Blast injuries also produced an unprecedented number of what orthopedists term "mangled extremities"—limbs with severe soft-tissue, bone, and often vascular injuries. These can be devastating, potentially mortal injuries, and whether to amputate is one of the most difficult decisions in orthopedic surgery. Military surgeons used to rely on civilian trauma criteria to guide their choices. Examination of their outcomes, however, revealed that those criteria were not reliable in this war. Possibly because the limb injuries were more extreme or more often combined with injuries to other organs, attempts to salvage limbs by following the criteria frequently failed, resulting in life-threatening blood loss, gangrene, and sepsis.

Late complications emerged as a substantial difficulty, as well. Surgeons began to see startling rates of pulmonary embolism and lower-extremity blood clots (deep venous thrombosis), for example, perhaps because of the severity of the extremity injuries and reliance on long-distance transportation of the wounded. Initial data showed that 5 percent of the wounded arriving at Walter Reed developed pulmonary emboli, resulting in two deaths. There was no obvious solution. Using anticoagulants—blood thinners—in patients with fresh wounds and in need of multiple procedures seemed unwise.

Mysteriously, injured soldiers from Iraq also brought an epidemic of infections from a multidrug-resistant bacteria called *Acinetobacter baumanii*. No such epidemic appeared among soldiers from Afghanistan, and whether the drug resistance was produced by antibiotic use or was already carried in the strains that had colonized troops in Iraq is unknown. Regardless, data from 442 medical evacuees seen at Walter Reed in 2004 showed that thirty-seven (8.4 percent) were culture-positive for *Acinetobacter*—a rate far higher than any previously experienced. The organism infected wounds, prostheses, and catheters in soldiers and spread to at least three other hospital patients. Later, medical evacuees from Iraq were routinely isolated on arrival and screened for the bacteria. Walter Reed, too, had to launch an effort to get health care personnel to be better about washing hands.

These were just the medical challenges. Other, equally pressing difficulties arose from the changing conditions of war. As the war converted from lightning-quick, highly mobile military operations to a more protracted, garrison effort, the CSHs had to adapt by converting to fixed facilities. In Baghdad, for example, medical personnel moved into the Ibn Sina hospital in the Green Zone. This shift brought increasing numbers of Iraqi civilians seeking care, and there was no overall policy about providing it. Some hospitals refused to treat civilians for fear of suicide bombers hiding among them in order to reach an American target. Others treated Iraqis but found themselves overwhelmed, particularly by pediatric patients, for whom they had limited personnel and few supplies.

Requests were made for additional staff members and resources at all levels. As the medical needs facing the military increased, however, the supply of medical personnel got tighter. Interest in signing up for military duty dropped precipitously. In 2004, according to the army, only fourteen other surgeons besides Murphy joined the reserves. Many surgeons were put on a second or extended deployment. But the numbers were not sufficient. Military urologists, plastic surgeons, and cardiothoracic surgeons were then tasked to fill some general surgeon positions. Planners began to contemplate ordering surgeons to take yet a third deployment. The Department of Defense announced that it would rely on improved financial incentives to attract more medical professionals. But the strategy did not succeed. The pay had never been competitive, and joined with the near certainty of leaving one's family for duty overseas and the dangerous nature of the work, it was not enough to encourage interest in entering military service. By the middle of 2005, the wars in Iraq and Afghanistan had stretched longer than American involvement in World War II—or in any war without a draft. In the absence of a draft, it has been extremely difficult for the nation's military surgical teams to maintain their remarkable performance.

Nonetheless, they have, at least thus far. At the end of 2006, medical teams were still saving an unbelievable 90 percent of soldiers wounded in battle. Military doctors continued to transform their strategies for the treatment of war casualties. They did so through a commitment to making a science of performance, rather than waiting for new discoveries. And they did it under extraordinarily demanding conditions and with heroic personal sacrifices.

One surgeon deserves particular recognition. Mark Taylor began his army service in 2001 as general surgeon at Fort Bragg's Womack Army Medical Center, in North Carolina, to fulfill the terms of the military scholarship that had allowed him to attend George Washington University Medical School several years before. He, like many others, was twice deployed to Iraq—first from February through May 2003 and then from August 2003 through winter the next year, as a member of the

782nd Forward Surgical Team. On March 20, 2004, outside Fallujah, four days from returning home, the forty-one-year-old surgeon was hit in a rocket-propelled-grenade attack while trying to make a phone call outside his barracks. Despite his team's efforts, he could not be revived. No doctor has paid a greater price.

PART II

Doing Right

Naked

There is an exquisite and fascinating scene in *Kandahar*, the 2001 movie set in Afghanistan under the Taliban regime, in which a male physician is asked to examine a female patient. They are separated by a dark blanketlike screen hung between them. Behind it, the woman is covered from head to foot by her burka. The two do not talk directly to each other. The patient's young son—he looks to be about six years old—serves as the go-between. She has a stomachache, he says.

"Does she throw up her food?" the doctor asks.

"Do you throw up your food?" the boy asks.

"No," the woman says, perfectly audibly, but the doctor waits as if he has not heard.

"No," the boy tells him.

For the purposes of examination, there is a two-inch circle cut in the screen. "Tell her to come closer," the doctor says. The boy does. She brings her mouth to the opening, and through it he looks inside. "Have her bring her eye to the hole," he says. And so the exam goes. Such, apparently, can be the demands of decency.

When I started in my surgical practice, I was not at all clear what my etiquette of examination should be. There are no clear standards in the United States, expectations are murky, and the topic can be fraught with hazards. Physical examination is deeply intimate, and the way a doctor deals with the naked body—particularly when the doctor is male and the patient female—inevitably raises questions of propriety and trust.

No one seems to have discovered the ideal approach. An Iraqi surgeon told me about the customs of physical examination in his home country. He said he feels no hesitation about examining female patients completely when necessary, but because a doctor and a patient of opposite sex cannot be alone together without eyebrows being raised, a family member will always accompany them for the exam. Women do not remove their clothes or change into a gown. Instead, only a small portion of the body is uncovered at any one time. A nurse, he said, is rarely asked to chaperone: if the doctor is female, it is not necessary, and if male, the family is there to ensure that nothing unseemly occurs.

In Caracas, according to a Venezuelan doctor I met, female patients virtually always have a chaperone for a breast or pelvic exam, whether the physician is male or female. "That way there are no mixed messages," the doctor said. The chaperone, however, must be a medical professional. So the family is sent out of the examination room, and a female nurse brought in. If a chaperone is unavailable or the patient refuses to allow one, the exam is not done.

A Ukrainian internist from Kiev told me that she has not heard of doctors there using a chaperone. I had to explain to her what a chaperone was. If a family member is present at an office visit, she said, he or she will be asked to leave. Both patient and doctor wear their uniforms—the patient a white examining gown, the doctor a white coat. Last names are always used. There is no effort at informality to muddy the occasion. These practices, she believes, are enough to solidify trust and preclude misinterpretation of the conduct of care.

A doctor, it appears, has a range of options.

In October 2003, I posted my clinic hours, and soon my first patients arrived to see me. For the first time, I realized, I was genuinely alone with patients. No attending physician supervising in the room or getting ready to come in; no bustle of emergency room personnel on the other side of a curtain. Just a patient and me. We'd sit down. We'd talk. I'd ask about whatever had occasioned the visit, about past medical problems, medications, the family and social history. Then the time would come to have a look.

There were, I will admit, some inelegant moments. I had an instinctive aversion to examination gowns. At our clinic they are made of either thin, ill-fitting cloth or thin, ill-fitting paper. They seem designed to leave patients exposed and cold. I decided to examine my patients while they were in their street clothes, for the sake of dignity. If a patient with gallstones wore a shirt she could untuck for the abdominal exam, this worked fine. But then I'd encounter a patient in tights and a dress, and the next thing I knew, I had her dress bunched up around her neck, her tights around her knees, and both of us wondering what the hell was going on. An exam for a breast lump one could manage, in theory: the woman could unhook her brassiere and lift or unbutton her shirt. But in practice, it just seemed weird. Even checking pulses could be a problem. Pant legs could not be pushed up high enough to check a femoral pulse. (The femoral artery is felt at the crease of the groin.) Try pulling them down over shoes, however, and . . . forget it. I finally began to have patients change into the damn gowns. (I haven't, however, asked men to do so nearly as often as women. I asked a female urologist friend of mine whether she had her male patients change into a gown for a genital or rectal examination. No, she said. Both of us just have them unzip and drop.)

As for having a chaperone present with female patients, I hadn't settled on a firm policy. I found that I always asked a medical assistant to come in for pelvic exams and generally didn't for breast exams. I was completely inconsistent about rectal exams.

I surveyed my colleagues about what they do and received a variety of answers. Many said they bring in a chaperone for all pelvic and rectal exams—"anything below the waist"—but only rarely for breast exams. Others have a chaperone for breast and pelvic exams but not for rectal exams. Some do not have a chaperone at all. Indeed, an obstetrician-gynecologist I talked to estimated that about half the male physicians in his department do not routinely use a chaperone. He himself detests the word *chaperone* because it implies that mistrust is warranted, but he offers to bring in an "assistant" for pelvic and breast exams. Few of his patients, however, find the presence of the assistant necessary after the first exam, he said. If the patient prefers to have her sister, boyfriend, or mother stay for the exam, he does not object—but he is under no illusion that a family chaperone offers protection against an accusation of misconduct. Instead, he relies on his reading of a patient to determine whether bringing in a nurse witness would be wise.

One of our residents, who was trained partly in London, said he found the selectivity here strange. "In Britain, I would never examine a woman's abdomen without a nurse present. But in the emergency room here, when I asked to have a nurse come in when I needed to do a rectal exam or check groin nodes on a woman, they thought I was crazy. 'Just go in there and do it!' they said." In England, he said, "if you need to do a breast or rectal exam or even check femoral pulses, especially on a young woman, you would be either foolish or stupid to do it without a chaperone. It doesn't take much—just one patient complaining, 'I came in with a foot pain and the doctor started diving around my groin,' and you could be suspended for a sexual harassment investigation."

Britain's standards are stringent: the General Medical Council, the Royal College of Physicians, and the Royal College of Obstetricians and Gynaecologists specify that a chaperone of the appropriate gender must be offered to all patients who undergo an "intimate examination" (that is, involving the breasts, genitalia, or rectum), irrespective of the gender of the patient or of the doctor. A chaperone must be present when a male physician performs an intimate examination of a female patient. The chaperone should be a female member of the medical team, and her name should be recorded in the notes. If the patient refuses a chaperone and the examination is not urgent, it is supposed to be deferred until it can be performed by a female physician.

In the United States, where we have no such guidelines, our patients have little idea of what to expect from us. To be sure, some minimal standards have been established. The Federation of State Medical Boards has spelled out that touching a patient's breasts or genitals for a purpose other than medical care is a sexual violation and a disciplinable offense. So are oral contact with a patient, encouraging a patient to masturbate in one's presence, and providing services in exchange for sexual favors. Sexual impropriety—which involves no touching but is no less proscribed—includes asking a patient for a date, criticizing a patient's sexual orientation, making sexual comments about the patient's body or clothing, and initiating discussion of one's own sexual experiences or fantasies. I can't say anyone taught me these boundaries in medical school, but I would like to think that no one needed to teach them.

The difficulty for doctors who behave properly is that medical exams remain inherently ambiguous. Any patient can be led to wonder: Did the doctor really need to touch me there? And when doctors simply inquire about patients' sexual history, can anyone be certain of the intent? The fact that all medical professionals have blushed or found their thoughts straying in unwanted directions during a patient visit reveals the potential for impropriety.

The tone of an office visit can turn on a single word, a

joke, a comment about a tattoo in an unexpected place. One surgeon told me of a young patient who expressed concern about a lump in her "boob." But when he used the same word in response, she became extremely uncomfortable and later made a complaint. A woman I know left her gynecologist after he let slip an offhand admiring comment about her tan lines during a pelvic exam.

The examination itself—the how and where of the touching—is, of course, the most potentially dicey territory. If a patient even begins to doubt the propriety of what a doctor is doing, something must not be right. So what then should our customs be?

There are many reasons to consider setting tighter, more uniform professional standards. One is to protect patients from harm. About 4 percent of the disciplinary orders that state medical boards issue against physicians are for sex-related offenses. One of every two hundred physicians is disciplined for sexual misconduct with patients sometime during his or her career. Some of these cases have involved such outrageous acts as having intercourse with patients during pelvic exams. The vast majority of cases involved male physicians and female patients, and virtually all occurred without a chaperone present. In one state, about a third of cases involved dating patients or sexual touching of them; two-thirds involved sexual impropriety or inappropriate touching short of sexual contact.

Clearer standards could also reduce false accusations against physicians. Chaperones in particular provide physicians with a stronger defense when such accusations are made. Inappropriate patient behavior might be averted, too. A 1994 study found that 72 percent of female medical students and 29 percent of male medical students experienced at least one instance of patient-initiated sexual behavior. Twelve percent of the females were sexually touched or grabbed by patients.

Yet, all this said, eliminating misconduct and accusations seems like the wrong priority to drive how doctors proceed when examining patients' bodies. The trouble is not that problems are rare (though the statistics suggest they are) or that total prevention of impropriety—zero tolerance—is impossible. It is that the measures required to achieve total prevention inevitably approach the Talibanesque and risk harming patients by discouraging complete and thorough examinations.

Instead, the most important reason to consider tightening standards of medical protocol is simply to improve trust and understanding between patients and doctors. The new informality of medicine—with white coats disappearing and patient and doctor sometimes on a first-name basis—has blurred boundaries that once guided us. If physicians are unsure about what the etiquette of the examination room should be, is it any surprise that patients are, too? Or that misinterpretations occur? We have jettisoned our old customs but we have not managed to replace them.

My father, a urologist, has thought carefully about how to avert such uncertainties. From the start, he told me, he felt the fragility of his standing as an outsider, an Indian immigrant practicing in our small southern Ohio town. In the absence of guidelines to reassure patients that what he does as a urologist is routine, he made painstaking efforts to avoid any question.

The process begins before the examination. He always arrives in a tie and white coat. He is courtly. Although he often knows patients socially and doesn't hesitate to speak with them about private matters (the subjects can range from impotence to sexual affairs), he keeps his language strictly medical. If a female patient must put on a gown, he steps out while she undresses. He makes a point of explaining what he is going to do during the examination and why. If the patient lies down and needs further unzipping or unbuttoning, he is careful not to help. He wears gloves even for abdominal examinations. If the patient is female or under eighteen years of age, he brings in a female nurse as a chaperone, whether the examination is "intimate" or not.

His approach works. He has a busy practice. There have been no unseemly rumors. I grew up knowing many of his patients, and they seemed to trust him completely.

I find, however, that some of his practices are not quite right for me. My patients are as likely to have problems above the waist as below, and having a chaperone present for a routine abdominal exam or an examination of enlarged lymph nodes under an arm seems absurd to me. I don't don gloves for nongenital exams, either. Nonetheless, I have tried to emulate the spirit of my father's visits—the decorum in language and attire, the respect for modesty, the precision of examination. And as I thought further about his example, I made changes: I now routinely bring in a female assistant not just for pelvic exams but also for female breast and rectal exams. "If it's all right, I'll go get Janice," I say. "She can be our chaperone."

IT IS UNSETTLING to find how little it takes to defeat success in medicine. You come as a professional equipped with expertise

and technology. You do not imagine that a mere matter of etiquette could foil you. But the social dimension turns out to be
as essential as the scientific—matters of how casual you
should be, how formal, how reticent, how forthright. Also:
how apologetic, how self-confident, how money-minded. In
this work against sickness, we begin not with genetic or cellu-
lar interactions, but with human ones. They are what make
medicine so complex and fascinating. How each interaction
is negotiated can determine whether a doctor is trusted,
whether a patient is heard, whether the right diagnosis is
made, the right treatment given. But in this realm there are no
perfect formulas.

Consider my chaperone solution, for example. A Man-
hattan friend in her thirties told me about seeing a dermatologist because of a mole she was worried about. The doctor was
in his sixties and perfectly professional. When it came time for
him to examine the mole and to check whether she had any
others under her threadbare examination gown, he brought in
a chaperone. This was, in theory, for her comfort and reassur-
ance. But the chaperone—a female aide who stood watching
as the dermatologist inspected my friend's body—only made
her feel more conspicuously on display.

"It was awkward," my friend told me. "The very idea of
a chaperone seems to shout: This is a highly charged situation,
and in order to avoid possible he-said, she-said litigation, this
nurse is going to stand silently and pointlessly in the corner. It
makes one feel *more* self-conscious and takes the weirdness
level up to Defcon 5. I felt like it turned a routine physical into
a silent Victorian melodrama."

So do male physicians make women more comfortable

with intimate examinations by involving a chaperone or not? My bet is that bringing an aide in helps more than it hurts. But we don't know; the study has never been done. And that itself is evidence of how much we've underestimated the importance and difficulty of human interactions in medicine. Everything from etiquette to economics, from anger to ethics can work its way into a seemingly routine office appointment. The relationships are deeply personal, involving promises and trust and hope, and this is what makes doing well as a clinician more than a matter of outcomes and statistics. One must also do right. How to do right by patients can be uncertain, sometimes overwhelmingly so. Do you bring in a chaperone or not? If, on your examination, you find a mole and think it is worrisome but a second opinion disagrees, do you reconsider your diagnosis or not? When you've tried several treatments and they fail, do you keep fighting or do you stop? Choices must be made. No choice will always be right. There are ways, however, to make our choices better.

What Doctors Owe

It was an ordinary Monday at the Middlesex County Superior Court in Cambridge, Massachusetts. Fifty-two criminal cases and a hundred and forty-seven civil cases were in session. In courtroom 6A, Daniel Kachoul was on trial on three counts of rape and three counts of assault. In courtroom 10B, David Santiago was on trial for cocaine trafficking and illegal possession of a deadly weapon. In courtroom 7B, a scheduling conference was being held for *Minihan v. Wallinger*, a civil claim of motor vehicle negligence. And next door, in courtroom 7A, Dr. Kenneth Reed faced charges of medical malpractice.

Reed was a Harvard-trained dermatologist with twenty-one years of experience, and he had never been sued for malpractice before. That day, he was being questioned about two office visits and a phone call that had taken place almost a decade earlier. Barbara Stanley, a fifty-eight-year-old woman, had been referred to him by her internist in the summer of 1996 about a dark warty nodule a quarter-inch wide on her left thigh. In the office, under local anesthesia, Reed shaved off the top for a biopsy. The pathologist's report came back a few days later, with a near-certain diagnosis of skin cancer—a malignant melanoma. At a follow-up appointment, Reed told Stanley that the growth would have to be completely removed. This would require taking a two-centimeter margin—almost an inch—of healthy skin beyond the lesion. He was worried about metastasis, and recommended that the procedure be done immediately, but she balked. The excision that he outlined on her leg would have been three inches across, and she couldn't believe that a procedure so disfiguring was necessary. She said that she had a friend who had been given a diagnosis of cancer erroneously and undergone unnecessary surgery. Reed pressed, though, and by the end of their discussion she allowed him to remove the visible tumor that remained on her thigh, only a half-inch excision, for a second biopsy. He, in turn, agreed to have another pathologist look at all the tissue and provide a second opinion.

To Reed's surprise, the new tissue specimen was found to contain no sign of cancer. And when the second pathologist, Dr. Wallace Clark, an eminent authority on melanoma, examined the first specimen he concluded that the initial cancer diagnosis was wrong. "I doubt if this is melanoma, but I cannot completely rule it out," his report said. Reed and Stanley spoke by phone in mid-September 1996 to go over the new findings.

None of this was in dispute; what was in dispute was what happened during the phone call. According to Stanley, Reed told her that she did not have a melanoma after all—the second opinion on the original biopsy "was negative"—and that no further surgery was required. Reed recalled the conversation differently. "I indicated to Barbara Stanley that Dr. Wallace Clark felt that this was a benign lesion called a Spitz nevus and that he could not be a 100 percent sure it was not a melanoma," he testified. "I also explained to her that in Dr. Clark's opinion this lesion had been adequately treated, that follow-up would be necessary, and that Dr. Clark did not feel that further surgery was critical. I also explained to Barbara Stanley that this was in conflict with the previous pathology report and that the most cautious way to approach this would be to allow me to [remove additional skin] for a two-centimeter margin." She became furious at him for the seeming error in his initial diagnosis, though, and told him that she didn't want more surgery. "At that point, I reemphasized to Barbara Stanley that at least she should come in for regular follow-up." She didn't want to return to see him. Indeed, she wrote him an angry letter afterward accusing him of mistreatment and refusing to pay his bill.

Two years later, the growth reappeared. Stanley went to another doctor, and this time the pathology report came back with a clear diagnosis: a deeply invasive malignant melanoma. A complete excision, she was told, should probably have been done the first time around. When she finally did undergo the more radical procedure, the cancer had spread to lymph nodes in her groin. She was started on a yearlong course of chemotherapy. Five months into it, she suffered a seizure. The cancer had spread to her brain and her left lung. She had a course of radiation. A few weeks after that, Barbara Stanley died.

But not before she had called a lawyer from her hospital bed. She found a full-page ad in the Yellow Pages for an attorney named Barry Lang, a specialist in medical malpractice cases, and he visited her at her bedside that very day. She told him that she wanted to sue Kenneth Reed. Lang took the case. Six years later, on behalf of Barbara Stanley's children, he stood up in a Cambridge courtroom and called Reed as his first witness.

MALPRACTICE SUITS ARE a feared, often infuriating, and common event in a doctor's life. (I have not faced a bona fide malpractice suit yet, but I know to expect one.) The average doctor in a high-risk practice like surgery or obstetrics is sued about once every six years. Seventy percent of the time, the suit is either dropped by the plaintiff or won by the doctor in court. But the cost of defense is high, and when doctors lose, the average jury verdict is half a million dollars. General surgeons pay anywhere from thirty thousand to three hundred thousand dollars a year in malpractice-insurance premiums, depending on the litigation climate of the state they work in; neurosurgeons and obstetricians pay upward of 50 percent more. This is a system that seems irrational to most physicians. Providing medical care is difficult. It involves the possibility of any of a thousand missteps, and no doctor will escape making some terrible ones. Lawsuits demanding six-figure sums for bad outcomes, therefore, seem mostly malicious to physicians—and even worse when no actual mistake is involved.

Every doctor, it seems, has a crazy-lawsuit story. My mother, a pediatrician, was once sued after a healthy two-month-old she had seen for a routine checkup died of sudden infant death syndrome a week later. The lawsuit alleged that she should have prevented the death, even though a defining characteristic of SIDS is that it occurs without warning. One of my colleagues performed lifesaving surgery to remove a woman's pancreatic cancer only to be sued years later because the woman developed a chronic pain in her arm; the patient blamed it, implausibly, on potassium that she received by IV during recovery from the surgery. I have a crazy-lawsuit story of my own. In 1990, while I was in medical school, I was standing at a crowded Cambridge bus stop when an elderly woman tripped on my foot and broke her shoulder. I gave her my phone number, hoping that she would call me and let me know how she was doing. She gave the number to a lawyer, and when he found out that it was a medical school exchange he tried to sue me for malpractice, alleging that I had failed to diagnose the woman's broken shoulder when I was trying to help her. (A marshal served me with a subpoena in physiology class.) When it became apparent that I was just a first-week medical student and hadn't been treating the woman, the court disallowed the case. The lawyer then sued me for half a million dollars, alleging that I'd run his client over with a bike. I didn't have a bike, but it took a year and a half—and fifteen thousand dollars in legal fees—to prove it.

My trial had taken place in the same courtroom as Reed's trial, and a shudder went through me when I recognized it.

Not everyone, however, sees the system the way doctors do, and I had come in an attempt to understand that gap in perspectives. In the courtroom gallery, I took a seat next to Ernie Browe, the son of Barbara Stanley. He was weary, he told me, after six years of excruciating delays. He worked for a chemistry lab in Washington State and had to take vacation time and use money from his savings to pay for hotels and flights—including for two trial dates that were postponed as soon as he arrived. "I wouldn't be here unless my mother asked me to, and she did before she died," he said. "She was angry, angry to have lost all those years because of Reed." He was glad that Reed was being called to account.

The dermatologist sat straight-backed and still in the witness chair as Lang fired questions at him. He tried not to get flustered. A friend of mine, a pediatric plastic surgeon who had had a malpractice suit go to trial, told me the instructions that his lawyer had given him for his court appearances: Don't wear anything flashy or expensive. Don't smile or joke or frown. Don't appear angry or uncomfortable, but don't appear overconfident or dismissive, either. How, then, are you supposed to look? Reed seemed to have settled on simply looking blank. He parsed every question for traps, but the strenuous effort to avoid mistakes only made him seem anxious and defensive.

"Wouldn't you agree," Lang asked, "that [melanoma] is very curable if it's excised before it has a chance to spread?" If a patient had asked this question, Reed would readily have said yes. But, with Lang asking, he paused, unsure.

"It's hypothetical," Reed said.

Lang was delighted with this sort of answer. Reed's

biggest problem, though, was that he hadn't kept notes on his mid-September phone conversation with Barbara Stanley. He could produce no corroboration for his version of events. And, as Lang often reminded the jury, plaintiffs aren't required to prove beyond a reasonable doubt that the defendant has committed malpractice. Lang needed ten of twelve jurors to think only that it was more likely than not.

"You documented a telephone conversation that you had with Barbara Stanley on August 31, isn't that correct?" Lang asked.

"That is correct."

"Your assistant documented a discussion that you had with Barbara Stanley on August 1, right?"

"That is correct."

"You documented a telephone call with Malden Hospital, correct?"

"That is correct."

"You documented a telephone conversation on September 6, when you gave Barbara Stanley a prescription for an infection, correct?"

"That is correct."

"So you made efforts and you had a habit of documenting patient interactions and telephone conversations, right?"

"That is correct."

Lang began to draw the threads together. "Exactly what Barbara Stanley needed, according to you, [was] a two-centimeter excision, right?"

"Which is what I instructed Ms. Stanley to do."

"Yet you did not tell Dr. Hochman"—Stanley's internist—"that she needed a two-centimeter excision, right?"

"That is correct."

"But you want this jury to believe you told Barbara Stanley?"

"I want this jury to believe the truth—which is that I told Barbara Stanley she needed a two-centimeter excision."

Lang raised his voice. "You should have told Barbara Stanley that, isn't that correct?" He all but called Reed a perjurer.

"I did tell Barbara Stanley, repeatedly!" Reed protested. "But she refused." Reed tried to keep his exasperation in check, while Lang did all he could to discredit him.

"In your entire career, Doctor, how many articles have you published in the literature?" Lang asked at another point.

"Three," Reed said.

Lang lifted his eyebrows and stood with his mouth agape for two beats. "In twenty years' time, you've published three articles?"

"Doctor, you do a lot of cosmetic medicine, isn't that true?" he later asked.

I could not tell whether the jury was buying Lang's insinuations. His examination made my skin crawl. I could picture myself on the stand being made to defend any number of cases in which things didn't turn out well and I hadn't got every last discussion down on paper. Lang was sixty years old, bald, short, and loud. He paced constantly and rolled his eyes at Reed's protestations. He showed no deference and little courtesy. He was almost a stereotype of a malpractice lawyer—except in one respect, and that was the reason I'd come to watch this particular trial: Barry Lang used to be a doctor.

For twenty-three years, he had a successful practice as an

orthopedic surgeon, with particular expertise in pediatric orthopedics. He'd even served as an expert witness on behalf of other surgeons. Then, in a turnabout, he went to law school, gave up his medical practice, and embarked on a new career suing doctors. Watching him, I wondered, had he come to a different understanding of doctors' accountability than the rest of us?

I WENT TO meet Lang at his office in downtown Boston, on the tenth floor of One State Street, in the heart of the financial district. He welcomed me warmly, and I found that we spoke more as fellow doctors than as potential adversaries. I asked why he had quit medicine to become a malpractice attorney. Was it for the money?

He laughed at the idea. Going into law "was a money disaster," he said. Starting out, he had expected at least some rewards. "I figured I'd get some cases, and if they were good the doctors would settle them quickly and get them out of the way. But no. I was incredibly naïve. No one ever settles before the actual court date. It doesn't matter how strong your evidence is. They always think they're in the right. Things can also change over time. And, given the choice of paying now or paying later, which would you rather do?"

He entered law practice, he said, because he thought he'd be good at it, because he thought he could help people, and because, after twenty-three years in medicine, he was burning out. "It used to be 'Two hip replacements today— yay!'" he recalled. "Then it became 'Two hip replacements today—ugh.'"

When I spoke to his wife, Janet, she said that his decision to change careers shocked her. From the day she met him, when they were undergraduates at Syracuse University, in New York, he'd never wanted to be anything other than a doctor. After medical school in Syracuse and an orthopedics residency at Temple University in Philadelphia, he had built a busy orthopedics practice in New Bedford, Massachusetts, and led a fulfilling and varied life. Even when he enrolled in night classes at Southern New England School of Law, a few blocks from his office, she didn't think anything of it. He was, as she put it, "forever going to school." One year, he took English literature classes at a local college. Another year, he took classes in Judaism. He took pilot lessons and before long was entering airplane aerobatics competitions. Law school, too, began as another pastime—"It was just for kicks," he said.

After he finished, though, he took the bar exam and got his license. He got certified as a public defender and took occasional cases defending indigent clients. He was fifty years old. He'd been in orthopedics practice long enough to have saved a lot of money, and law began to seem much more interesting than medicine. In July 1997 he handed his practice over to his startled partners, "and that was the end of it," he said.

He figured that the one thing he could offer was his medical expertise, and he tried to start his legal practice by defending physicians. But because he had no experience, the major law firms that dealt with malpractice defense wouldn't take him, and the malpractice insurers in the state wouldn't send him cases. So he rented a small office and set up shop as a malpractice attorney for patients. He sunk several thousand dollars a month into ads on television and in the phone book, dubbing himself "the Law Doctor." Then the phone calls came. Five years into his new career, his cases finally began going to trial. This was his eighth year as a malpractice attorney, and he had won settlements in at least thirty cases. Eight others had gone to trial, and he had won most of them, too. Two weeks before the Reed trial, he won a $400,000 jury award for a woman whose main bile duct was injured during gallbladder surgery and required several reconstructive operations. (Lang got more than a third of that award. Under Massachusetts state law, attorneys get up to 40 percent of the first $150,000, 33.3 percent of the next $150,000, 30 percent of the next $200,000, and 25 percent of anything over half a million.) Lang has at least sixty cases pending. If he had any money troubles, they are over now.

Lang said that he receives ten to twelve calls a day, mostly from patients or their families, with some referrals from lawyers who don't do malpractice. He turns most of them away. He wants a good case, and a good case has to have two things, he said. "Number one, you need the doctor to be negligent. Number two, you need the doctor to have caused damage." Many of the cases fail on both counts. "I had a call from one guy. He says, 'I was waiting in the emergency room for four hours. People were taken ahead of me, and I was really sick.' I say, 'Well, what happened as a result of that?' 'Nothing, but I shouldn't have to wait for four hours.' Well, that's ridiculous."

Some callers have received negligent care but suffered little harm. In a typical scenario, a woman sees her doctor about a lump in her breast and is told not to worry about it. Still concerned, she sees another doctor, gets a biopsy, and learns that she has cancer. "So she calls me up, and she wants to sue the first doctor," Lang said. "Well, the first doctor was negligent. But what are the damages?" She got a timely diagnosis and treatment. "The damages are nothing."

I asked him how great the prospective damages had to be to make the effort worth his while. "It's a gut thing," he said. His expenses on a case are typically forty to fifty thousand dollars. So he would almost never take, say, a dental case. "Is a jury going to give me fifty thousand dollars for the loss of a tooth? The answer is no." The bigger the damages, the better. As another attorney told me, "I'm looking for a phone number"—damages worth seven figures.

Another consideration is how the plaintiff will come across to jurors. Someone may have a great case on paper, but Lang listens with a jury in mind. Is this person articulate enough? Will he or she seem unreasonable or strange to others? Indeed, a number of malpractice attorneys I spoke to confirmed that the nature of the plaintiff, not just of the injury, was a key factor in the awarding of damages. Vernon Glenn, a highly successful trial attorney from Charleston, South Carolina, told me, "The ideal client is someone who matches the social, political, and cultural template of where you are." He told me about a case he had in Lexington County, South Carolina—a socially conservative, devoutly Christian county that went 72 percent for George W. Bush in the 2004 election and produces juries unsympathetic to malpractice lawyers. But his plaintiff was a white, Christian female in her thirties with three young children who had lost her husband—a hard-working, thirty-nine-year-old truck mechanic who loved NASCAR, had voted Republican for the past twenty years, and had built the addition to their country home himself—to a medical error. During routine gallbladder surgery, doctors caused a bowel injury that they failed to detect (his wife called several times about his worsening pain after he was discharged home from the hospital, but she was told to just give him more pain medication) until he collapsed and died. The woman was articulate and attractive but not so good-looking as to put off a jury. She wasn't angry or vengeful but was visibly grieving and in need of help. If the family hadn't spoken English, if the husband had a long history of mental illness or alcoholism or cigarette smoking, if they'd been involved in previous lawsuits or had a criminal record, Glenn might not have taken the case. As it was, "she was darn close to the perfect client," he said. The day before trial, the defendants settled for $2.4 million.

Out of sixty callers a week, Barry Lang might take the next step with two and start reviewing the medical records for hard evidence of negligent care. Many law firms have a nurse or a nurse practitioner on staff to do the initial review. But Lang himself gathers all the records, arranges them chronologically, and goes through them page by page.

There is a legal definition of negligence ("when a doctor has breached his or her duty of care"), but I wanted to know his practical definition of the term. Lang said that if he finds an error that resulted in harm and the doctor could have avoided it, then, as far as he is concerned, the doctor was negligent.

To most doctors, this is an alarming definition. Given the difficulty of many cases—unclear diagnoses, delicate operations—we all cause serious complications that might have been avoided. I told Lang about a few patients of mine: a man with severe bleeding after laparoscopic liver surgery, a patient who was left permanently hoarse after thyroid surgery, a woman whose breast cancer I failed to diagnose for months. All were difficult cases. But in looking back on them, I also now see ways in which I could have done better. Would he sue me? If he could show a jury how I might have avoided harm and if the damages were substantial, "I would sue you in a flash," he said. But what if I have a good record among surgeons, with generally excellent outcomes and conscientious care? That wouldn't matter, he said. The only thing that matters is what I did in the case in question. It's like driving a car, he explained—I could have a perfect driving record, but if one day I run a red light and hit a child, then I am negligent, he said.

Lang insists that he is not on a crusade against doctors. He faced three malpractice lawsuits himself when he was a surgeon. One involved an arthroscopy that he performed on a young woman with torn cartilage in her knee from a sports injury. Several years later, he said, she sued because she developed arthritis in the knee—a known, often unavoidable outcome. Against his wishes, the insurer settled with the patient for what Lang called "nuisance money"—five thousand dollars or so—because it was cheaper than fighting the suit in court.

In another case, a manual laborer with a wrist injury that caused numbness in three fingers sued because Lang's attempted repair made the numbness worse and left him unable to work. Lang said that he'd warned the patient that this was a high-risk surgery. When he got in, he found the key nerves encased in a thick scar. Freeing them was exceedingly difficult— "like trying to peel Scotch tape off wallpaper," he said—and some nerve fibers were unavoidably pulled off. But the insurer wasn't certain that the argument would prevail at trial and settled for $300,000. Both cases seemed unmerited, and Lang found them as exasperating as any other doctor would.

The third case, however, was the result of a clear error, and although it took place two decades ago, it still bothers him. "I could have done more," he told me. The patient was a man in his sixties whom Lang had scheduled for a knee replacement. A few days before the surgery, the man came to Lang's office complaining of pain in his calf. Lang considered the possibility of a deep-vein thrombosis—a blood clot in the leg—but dismissed it as unlikely and ordered no further testing. The patient did have a D.V.T., though, and when the clot dislodged two days later, it traveled to his lungs and killed him. Lang's insurer settled the case for about $400,000.

"If I had been on the plaintiff's side, would I have taken that case against me?" he said. "Yes."

Being sued was "devastating," Lang recalled. "It's an awful feeling. No physician purposely harms his patient." Yet he insists that, even at the time, he was philosophical about the cases. "Being sued, although it sort of sucks the bottom out of you, you have to understand that it's also the cost of doing business. I mean, everybody at some time in his life is negligent, whether he's a physician, an auto mechanic, or an accountant. Negligence occurs, and that's why you have insurance. If you leave the oven on at home and your house catches fire, you're negligent. It doesn't mean you're a criminal." In his view, the public has a reasonable expectation: if a physician causes someone serious harm from substandard

care or an outright mistake, he or she should be held account-
able for the consequences.

The three cases that Lang faced as a doctor seemed to
me to epitomize the malpractice debate. Two of the three
lawsuits against him appeared unfounded, and, whatever Lang
says now, the cost to our system in money and confidence is
nothing to dismiss. Yet one of them concerned a genuine error that cost a man his life. In such cases, don't doctors owe
something to patients and their families?

BILL FRANKLIN IS a physician I know who has practiced at
Massachusetts General Hospital, in Boston, for more than
four decades. He is an expert in the treatment of severe, life-
threatening allergies. He is also a father. Years ago, his son Peter, who was then a second-year student at Boston University
School of Medicine, called to say that he was feeling sick. He
had sweats and a cough and felt exhausted. Franklin had him
come to his office and looked him over. He didn't find any obvious explanation for his son's symptoms, so he had him get a
chest X-ray. Later that day, the radiologist called. "We've got
big trouble," he told Franklin. The X-ray showed a tumor filling Peter's chest, compressing his lungs from the middle and
pushing outward. It was among the largest the radiologist had
encountered.

After he had pulled himself together, Franklin called Peter at home to give him and his young wife the frightening
news. They had two children and a small house, with a
kitchen that they were in the midst of renovating. Their lives

came to a halt. Peter was admitted to the hospital and a biopsy showed that he had Hodgkin's lymphoma. He was put on high-dose radiation therapy, with a beam widened to encompass his chest and neck. Still, Peter was determined to return to school. He scheduled his radiation sessions around his coursework, even after they paralyzed his left diaphragm and damaged his left lung, leaving him unable to breathe normally.

The tumor proved too large and extensive for a radiation cure. Portions of it continued to grow, and it spread to two lymph nodes in Peter's lower abdomen. The doctors told his father that it was one of the worst cases they had seen. Peter was going to need several months of chemotherapy. It would make him sick and leave him infertile, but, they said, it should work.

Franklin couldn't understand how the tumor had got so large under everyone's eyes. Thinking back on Peter's care over the years, he remembered that four years earlier Peter's wisdom teeth had been removed. The surgery had been performed under general anesthesia, with an overnight stay at MGH, and a chest X-ray would have been taken. Franklin had one of the radiologists pull the old X-ray and take a second look. The mass was there, the radiologist told him. What's more, the original radiologist who had reviewed Peter's chest X-ray had seen it. "Further evaluation of this is recommended," the four-year-old report said. But the Franklins had never been told. The oral surgeon and the surgical resident had both written in Peter's chart that the X-ray was normal.

If the tumor had been treated then, Peter would almost certainly have been cured with radiation alone, and with considerably less-toxic doses. Now it seemed unlikely that he'd finish medical school, if he survived at all. Bill Franklin was beside himself. How could this have happened—to one of MGH's own, no less? How would Peter's wife and children be supported?

Thousands of people in similar circumstances file malpractice lawsuits to get answers to such questions. That's not what Bill Franklin wanted to do. The doctors involved in his son's case were colleagues and friends, and he was no fan of the malpractice system. He had himself been sued. He'd had a longtime patient with severe asthma whom he had put on steroids to ease her breathing during a bad spell. Her asthma had improved, but the high steroid doses produced a prolonged psychosis, and she had to be hospitalized. The lawsuit alleged that Franklin had been negligent in putting her on steroids, given the risks of the medication, and that he was therefore financially responsible for the aftermath. Franklin was outraged. She'd had a life-threatening problem, and he'd given her the best care he could.

Now, for Peter's sake, he decided to see the hospital director. He asked for a small investigation into how the mistake had been made and how it might be prevented in the future; he also wanted to secure financial support for Peter's family. The director told him that he couldn't talk to him about the matter. He should get a lawyer, he said. Was there no other way? Franklin wanted to know. There wasn't.

This is where we in medicine have failed. When something bad happens in the course of care and a patient and family want to know whether it was unavoidable or due to a terrible mistake, where are they to turn? Most people turn first to the doctors involved. Doctors have an ethical responsibility to tell patients when an error has harmed them. But what if they aren't responsive—what if they seem to be worrying more about a lawsuit than about the patient—or what if their explanations don't sound quite right? People often call an attorney just to get help in finding out what happened.

"Most people aren't sure what they're coming to me for," Vernon Glenn, the South Carolina trial attorney, told me. "The tipoff is often from nurses saying, 'This was just wrong. This should never have happened.'" The families ask him to have a look at the medical files. If the loss or injury is serious, he has an expert review the files. "More often than you would think, we'll say, 'Here's what happened. We don't think it's a case.' And they'll say, 'At least we know what happened now.'"

Malpractice attorneys are hardly the most impartial assessors of care, but medicine has offered no genuine alternative—because we physicians are generally unwilling to be held financially responsible for the consequences of our mistakes. Indeed, the one argument that has persuaded many doctors to be more forthright about mistakes is that doing so might make patients less likely to sue.

Yet, when the tables are turned and someone close to a doctor is hurt by a medical mistake, our views seem to shift. In a recent national survey, physicians and nonphysicians were given the following case: A surgeon orders an antibiotic for a sixty-seven-year-old man undergoing surgery, failing to notice that the patient's chart says that he is allergic to the drug. The mistake is not caught until after the antibiotic is given, and, despite every effort, the patient dies as a result. What should be done? Unlike 50 percent of the lay public, almost none of the physicians believed the surgeon should lose his license. But 55 percent of the physicians said that they would sue the surgeon for malpractice.

That's what Bill Franklin, with some trepidation, decided to do. Lawyer friends warned him that he might have to leave his position on staff if things didn't go well. He loved the hospital and his practice; Peter's oral surgeon was a friend. But his son had been harmed, and he felt that Peter and his young family were entitled to compensation for all that they had lost and suffered. Peter himself was against suing. He was afraid that a lawsuit might so antagonize his doctors that they would not treat him properly. But he was persuaded to go along with it.

At first, the Franklins were told that no lawyer would take the case. The error had been made four years earlier, and this put it beyond the state's three-year statute of limitations. As in most other states at the time, one could not file a civil claim for an action long in the past—never mind that Peter didn't learn about the error until it was too late. Then they found a young Boston trial attorney named Michael Mone, who took the case all the way to the Massachusetts Supreme Court and, in 1980, won a change in the law. *Franklin v. Massachusetts General Hospital et al.* ruled that such time limits must start with the discovery of harm, and the precedent stands today. The change allowed the case to proceed.

The trial was held in 1983, in the town of Dedham, in the same courthouse where, six decades earlier, the anarchists Sacco and Vanzetti had been convicted of murder. "I don't remember much about the trial—I've blocked it out," Bev Franklin, Peter's mother, says. "But I remember the room. And I remember Michael Mone saying those words we'd been waiting so long to hear: 'Ladies and gentlemen, this young

man had a time bomb ticking in his chest. And for four years—
four years—the doctors did nothing.' " The trial took four days.
The jury found in favor of Peter and awarded him $600,000.

Bill Franklin says that he never experienced any negative
repercussions at the hospital. His colleagues seemed to understand, and Peter's doctors did their very best for him. At the
end of a long year, after six full cycles of chemotherapy, the
lymph nodes in Peter's chest continued to harbor residual cancer. He was given a new chemotherapy regimen, which so
weakened his immune system that he almost died of a viral
lung infection. He was in the hospital for weeks and was finally forced to take a leave from school. The virus left him
short of breath whenever he did anything more strenuous
than climb half a flight of stairs, and with burning nerve pain
in his feet. His marriage slowly disintegrated; a disaster can either draw people together or pull them apart, and this one
pulled Peter and his wife apart.

Yet Peter survived. He eventually completed medical
school and decided to go into radiology. To everyone's surprise, he was rejected by his top-choice residency programs. A
dean at Boston University called the chairman of radiology at
one of the programs to find out why. "This guy's a maverick!
He's suing doctors!" was the reply. The dean told the chairman Peter's story and then asked, "If this was your son, what
would you do?" Peter got in after that. He chose Boston University's program and, when he finished, he was asked to join
the staff there. Soon, he was made a division chief. He remar-
ried and is now a fifty-eight-year-old expert on orthopedic imaging, with a brush mustache, a graying thatch of hair, and
chronic lung and liver troubles from his chemotherapy. In

2000, he started a teleradiology group that now interprets scans for 150 centers across the country. He is also a special consultant to professional sports teams, including the San Diego Chargers and the Chicago Bears.

He says that his ordeal has made him exceedingly careful in his work. He has set up a review committee to find and analyze errors. Nonetheless, the single biggest budget item for his group is malpractice insurance. As it happens, the most common kind of malpractice case in the country involves allegations that doctors have made the sort of error that Peter once faced—a missed or delayed diagnosis. I asked him how he felt about being responsible for a lawsuit that had made it easier to sue for such claims. He winced and paused to consider his answer.

"I think the malpractice system has run amok," he finally said. "I don't think that my little experience has anything to do with it—the system is just so rampant with problems. But if you're damaged, you're damaged. If we screw up, I think we should eat it." Wasn't he contradicting himself? No, he said; the system was the contradiction. Few of the people who deserve compensation actually get any. His case was unusual in that he did get compensated, and even so, it involved a seven-year struggle before all the appeals and challenges were dismissed. At the same time, too many undeserving patients sue, imposing enormous expense and misery. The system, as he sees it, is fundamentally perverse.

THE PARADOX AT the heart of medical care is that it works so well, and yet never well enough. It routinely gives people years of health that they otherwise wouldn't have had. Death rates from heart disease have plummeted by almost two-thirds since the 1950s. Risk of death from stroke has fallen more than 80 percent. The cancer survival rate is now 70 percent. But these advances have required drugs and machines and operations and, most of all, decisions that can as easily damage people as save them. It's precisely because of our enormous success that people are bound to wonder what went wrong when we fail.

As a surgeon, I will perform about 350 operations in the next year—everything from emergency repair of strangulated groin hernias to removal of thyroid cancers. For six, maybe eight patients—roughly 2 percent—things will not go well. They will develop life-threatening bleeding. Or I will damage a critical nerve. Or I will make a wrong diagnosis. Whatever Hippocrates may have said, sometimes we do harm. Studies of serious complications find that usually about half are unavoidable, and in such cases I might be able to find some solace in knowing this. But in the other half I will have done something wrong, and my mistake may change someone's life forever. Society is still searching for an adequate way to understand these instances. Are doctors who make mistakes villains? No, because then we all are. But we are tainted by the harm we cause.

I watch a lot of baseball, and I often find myself thinking about the third baseman's job. In a season, a third baseman will have about as many chances to throw a man out as I will to operate on people. The very best (players like Mike Lowell, Hank Blalock, Bill Mueller) do this perfectly almost every time. But 2 percent of the time even they drop the ball or throw it over the first baseman's head. No one playing a full season fails to make stupid errors. When a player does, the fans hoot and jeer. If his error costs the game, the hooting will turn to yelling. Imagine, though, that if every time Mike Lowell threw and missed, the error cost or damaged the life of someone you cared about. One error leaves an old man with a tracheostomy; another puts a young woman in a wheelchair; another leaves a child brain-damaged for the rest of her days. His teammates would still commiserate, but the rest of us? Some would want to rush the field howling for Lowell's blood. Others would see all the saves he's made and forgive him his failures. Nobody, though, would see him in quite the same light again. And nobody would be happy to have the game go on as if nothing had happened. We'd want him to show sorrow, to take responsibility. We'd want the people he injured to be helped in a meaningful way.

This is our situation in medicine, and litigation has proved to be a singularly unsatisfactory solution. It is expensive, drawn out, and painfully adversarial. It helps very few people. Ninety-eight percent of American families that are hurt by medical errors don't sue. They are unable to find lawyers who think they would make good plaintiffs, or they are simply too daunted. Of those who do sue—about fifty-five thousand a year—most will lose. In the end, fewer than one in a hundred deserving families receive any money. The rest get nothing: no help, not even an apology. And only the worst is brought out in all of us.

THERE IS AN alternative approach, which was developed for people who have been injured by vaccines. Vaccines protect tens of millions of children, but every year one in ten thousand or so is harmed by side effects. Between 1980 and 1986, personal-injury lawyers filed damage claims in U.S. courts valued at more than $3.5 billion against doctors and manufacturers. When they began to win, vaccine prices jumped and some manufacturers got out of the business. Vaccine stockpiles dwindled. Shortages appeared. So Congress stepped in. American vaccines now carry a seventy-five-cent surcharge (about 15 percent of total costs), which goes into a fund for children who are injured by them. The program does not waste effort trying to sort those who are injured through negligence from those who are injured through bad luck. An expert panel has enumerated the known injuries from vaccines, and, if you have one, the fund provides compensation for medical and other expenses. If you're not satisfied, you can sue in court. But few have. Since 1988, the program has paid out a total of $1.5 billion to injured patients. Because these costs are predictable and evenly distributed, vaccine manufacturers have not only returned to the market but produced new vaccines, including ones against hepatitis, chicken pox, and cervical cancer. The program also makes the data on manufacturers public—who got sued and for what—whereas legal settlements in medical cases are virtually always sealed from view. The system has flaws, but it has helped far more people than the courts would have.

The central problem with any system remotely as fair and efficient as this one is that, applied more broadly, it would be overwhelmed with cases. Even if each doctor had just one injured and deserving patient a year (a highly optimistic assumption), complete compensation would exceed the cost of providing universal health coverage in America. To be practical, the system would have to have firm and perhaps arbitrary-seeming limits on eligibility as well as on compensation. New Zealand has settled for a system like this. For some thirty years, it has offered compensation for medical injuries that are rare (occurring in less than 1 percent of cases) and severe (resulting in death or prolonged disability). As with America's vaccine fund, there is no attempt to sort the victims of error from the victims of bad luck. For those who qualify, the program pays for lost income, medical needs, and, if there's a permanent disability, an additional lump sum for the suffering endured. Payouts are made within nine months of filing. There are no mammoth, random windfalls, as there are in our system, but the public sees the amounts as reasonable and there's no clamor to send these cases back to the courts.

The one defense of our malpractice system is that it has civilized the passions that arise when a doctor has done a devastating wrong. It may not be a rational system, but it does give people with the most heartbreaking injuries a means to fight. Every once in a while, it extracts enough money from a doctor to provide not just compensation but the satisfaction of a resounding punishment, fair or not. And although it does nothing for most plaintiffs, people whose loved ones have suffered complications do not then riot in hospital hallways, as clans have done in some countries.

Every few years in the United States, there is a flurry of efforts to "reform" our malpractice system. More than half of American states have enacted caps on the amount of money that juries can award someone who has been injured by a doctor. But no such ceiling will make the system fairer or less frustrating for either doctors or patients. It simply puts an arbitrary limit on payments so that doctors' insurance premiums might, at least temporarily, be more affordable.

Cap or no cap, I will pay more than half a million dollars in premiums in the next ten years. I would much rather see that money placed in a fund for my patients who suffer complications from my care, even if the fund cannot be as generous as we'd like it to be. There's no real chance of this happening right now, though. For the moment, we must make do with what we have.

IN COURTROOM 7A of the Edward J. Sullivan Courthouse in Cambridge, after seven years of litigation, more than twenty thousand dollars in payments to medical experts, the procurement of bailiffs, court reporters, a judge, and $250-an-hour defense attorneys, time on an overloaded court schedule, and the commandeered lives of fourteen jurors for almost two weeks, Barry Lang stood behind a lectern to make his closing argument on behalf of the estate of Barbara Stanley. For the first time during the trial, Lang stopped his constant pacing. He spoke slowly and plainly. The story he told seemed lucid and coherent. In that fateful telephone conversation, he argued, Reed failed to offer Stanley the option of a more radical skin excision that might have saved her life. "Dr. Reed is not a criminal," Lang told the jury. "But he was negligent, and his negligence was a key factor in causing Barbara Stanley's death."

Lang, however, did not have an open-and-shut case. As Reed's lawyer argued to the jury in his closing, Reed had been faced with a difficult medical problem: pathologists who contradicted each other about whether the first biopsy showed skin cancer, a second biopsy that failed to settle the issue, and a distrusting patient who was angry with him for doing too much in the first place. It was far from certain—then or in hindsight—that doing a more radical excision would have helped. Under the microscope, the margins of the tissue Reed had excised around Stanley's tumor were clear of disease. His experts had therefore testified that the cancer had likely already spread and that taking yet more tissue would not have changed that. Furthermore, Reed steadfastly insisted that he had offered Stanley the option of a more radical excision from the beginning.

When the lawyers finished their closings, Judge Kenneth Fishman gave the jury its instructions. Stanley's son, Ernie Browe, sat in the front row of the gallery on one side, and Kenneth Reed sat a row back on the other. Both looked drained. By the time the judge finished, it was late in the afternoon, and to Browe and Reed's disappointment, he dismissed everyone for the day. Both had expected to know the outcome by the day's end.

The next morning, the jury finally began its deliberations. Just before noon, the court officer announced that a verdict had been reached: Dr. Kenneth Reed was not negligent in his care of Barbara Stanley. Stanley's son slumped in his seat, looked down at the floor, and did not move for a long while. Barry Lang promptly stood up to put away his papers. "It was a tough case," he said. Reed was not there to hear the verdict. He had been in his office all morning, seeing patients.

Piecework

To become a doctor, you spend so much time in the tunnels of preparation—head down, trying not to screw up, just going from one day to the next—that it is a shock to find yourself at the other end, with someone shaking your hand and offering you a job. But the day comes. Mine came as I was finishing my eighth and final year as a resident in surgery. I had got a second interview for a surgical staff position at the hospital in Boston where I had trained. It was a great job—I'd be able to do general surgery, but I'd also get to specialize in surgery for certain tumors that interested me. On the appointed day, I put on my fancy suit and took a seat in the wood-paneled office of the chairman of surgery. He sat down opposite me and then he told me the job was mine. "Do you want it?" Yes, I said, a little startled. The position, he explained, came with a guaranteed salary for three years. After that, I would be on my own: I'd make what I brought in from my patients and would pay my own expenses. So, he went on, how much should they pay me?

After all those years of being told how much I would either pay (about forty thousand dollars a year for medical school) or get paid (about forty thousand dollars a year in residency), I was stumped. "How much do the surgeons usually make?" I asked.

He shook his head. "Look," he said, "you tell me what you think is an appropriate income to start with until you're on your own. If it's reasonable that's what we'll pay you." He gave me a few days to think about it.

MOST PEOPLE GAUGE what they deserve to be paid by what others are paid for doing the same work, so I tried asking various members of the surgical staff. These turned out to be awkward conversations. I'd pose my little question, and they'd start mumbling as if their mouths were full of crackers. I tried all kinds of formulations. Maybe they could tell me how much take-home pay would be if one did, say, eight major operations a week? Or how much they thought I should ask for? Nobody would give me a number.

Most people are squeamish about saying how much they earn, but in medicine the situation seems especially fraught. Doctors aren't supposed to be in it for the money, and the more concerned a doctor seems to be about making money the more suspicious people become about the care being provided. (That's why the good doctors on TV hospital dramas drive old cars and live in ramshackle apartments, while the bad doctors wear bespoke suits.) During our hundred-hour-a-week, just-over-minimum-wage residencies, we all take a self-righteous pleasure in hinting to people about how hard we work and how little we earn. Settled into practice a few years later, doctors clam up. Since the early 1980s, public surveys have indicated that two-thirds of Americans believe doctors are "too interested in making money." Yet the health care system, as I soon discovered, requires doctors to give inordinate attention to matters of payment and expenses.

To get a sense of the numbers involved, I asked our physician group's billing office for a copy of its "master fee schedule," which lists what various insurers pay our doctors for the care they provide. It has twenty-four columns across the top, one for each of the major insurance plans, and, running down the side, a row for every service a doctor can bill for. Our current version goes on for more than six hundred pages. Everything's in there, with a dollar amount attached. For those who have Medicare, the government insurance program for the elderly—its payments are near the middle of the range—an office visit for a new patient with a "low complexity" problem (service No. 99203) pays $77.29. A visit for a "high complexity" problem (service No. 99205) pays $151.92. Setting a dislocated shoulder (service No. 23650) pays $275.70. Removing a bunion: $492.35. Removing an appendix: $621.31. Removing a lung: $1,662.34. The best-paid service on the list? Surgical reconstruction for a baby born without a diaphragm: $5,366.98. The lowest-paying? Trimming a patient's nails ("any number"): $10.15. The hospital collects separately for any costs it incurs.

The notion of a schedule like this, with services and fees laid out à la carte like a menu from Chili's, may seem odd. In fact, it's rooted in ancient history. Doctors have been paid on a piecework basis since at least the Code of Hammurabi; in Babylon during the eighteenth century B.C., a surgeon got ten shekels for any lifesaving operation he performed (only two shekels if the patient was a slave). The standardized fee schedule, though, is a thoroughly modern development. In the 1980s, insurers, both public and private, began to agitate for a more "rational" schedule of physician payments. For decades, they had been paying physicians according to what were called "usual, customary, and reasonable fees." This was more or less whatever doctors decided to charge. Not surprisingly, some of the charges began to rise considerably. There were some egregious distortions. For instance, fees for cataract surgery (which could reach six thousand dollars in 1985) had been set when the operation typically took two to three hours. When new technologies allowed ophthalmologists to do it in thirty minutes, the fees didn't change. Billings for this one operation grew to consume 4 percent of Medicare's budget. In general, payments for doing procedures had far outstripped payments for diagnoses. In the mid-eighties, doctors who spent an hour making a complex and lifesaving diagnosis were paid forty dollars; for spending an hour doing a colonoscopy and excising a polyp, they received more than six hundred dollars.

This was, the federal government decided, unacceptable. The system discouraged good primary care and corrupted specialty care. So the government determined that payments ought to be commensurate with the amount of work involved. The principle was simple and sensible; putting it into practice was another matter. In 1985, William Hsiao, a Harvard economist, was commissioned to measure the exact amount of work involved in each of the tasks doctors perform. It must have seemed a quixotic assignment, something like being asked to measure the exact amount of anger in the world. But Hsiao came up with a formula. Work, he determined, was a function of time spent, mental effort and judgment, technical skill and physical effort, and stress. He put together a large team that interviewed and surveyed thousands of physicians from some two dozen specialties. They analyzed what was involved in everything from forty-five minutes of psychotherapy for a patient with panic attacks to a hysterectomy for a woman with cervical cancer.

They determined that the hysterectomy takes about twice as much time as the session of psychotherapy, 3.8 times as much mental effort, 4.47 times as much technical skill and physical effort, and 4.24 times as much risk. The total calculation: 4.99 times as much work. Estimates and extrapolations were made in this way for thousands of services. (Cataract surgery was estimated to involve slightly less work than a hysterectomy.) Overhead and training costs were factored in. Eventually, Hsiao and his team arrived at a relative value for every single thing doctors do. Some specialists were outraged by particular estimates. But Congress set a multiplier to convert the relative values into dollars, the new fee schedule was signed into law, and in 1992 Medicare started paying doctors accordingly. Private insurers followed shortly thereafter (although they applied somewhat different multipliers, depending on the deals they struck with local physicians).

There is a certain arbitrariness to the result. Who can really say whether a hysterectomy is more labor-intensive than cataract surgery? A subsequent commission has reexamined and recalibrated the relative values for more than six thousand different services. Such toil will no doubt continue in perpetuity. But the system has been accepted—more or less.

EVEN WITH THE fee schedule in front of me, I had a hard time figuring out how much I'd earn. My practice would primarily involve office visits, some general surgery (appendectomies, gallbladder removals, bowel and breast surgery), and—given my interest in endocrine tumors—a lot of thyroid and adrenal surgery. Each of these procedures pays between six hundred and eleven hundred dollars, and I could expect to do eight or so a week. Assuming I worked forty-eight weeks, it seemed that I could make a flabbergasting half-million dollars a year. But then I'd have to spend thirty-one thousand dollars a year on malpractice insurance and eighty thousand dollars a year to rent office and clinic space. I'd have to buy computers and other office equipment and hire a secretary and a medical assistant or a nurse. The department of surgery deducts 19.5 percent for its overhead. Then there are the patients who don't have insurance and can't afford to pay—15 percent of Americans are uninsured, and like many other doctors, I believe we're obligated to care for such patients insofar as we can. Furthermore, even when patients are insured, some insurance companies pay far less than others. Studies also indicate that insurers find a reason to reject payment for up to 30 percent of the bills they receive.

Roberta Parillo is a financial-disaster specialist for doctors who is called in by physician groups or hospitals when they suddenly find that they can't make ends meet. ("I fix messes" was the way she put it to me.) She started out in graduate school in American literature ("I was going to be a writer") but when that didn't pan out, she began working with a group of Connecticut doctors, helping them figure out insurance forms. She's now in her fifties, living on airplanes and in hotels and still doing much the same. At the time I spoke to her, she was in Pennsylvania, trying to figure out where things had gone wrong for a struggling hospital. In previous months, she'd been to Mississippi to help a group of a 125 physicians who found they were in debt, to Washington, D.C., where a physician group was worried about its survival, and to New England (she didn't want to say exactly where), for a big anesthesiology department that had lost fifty million dollars. She'd turned away a dozen other clients. It's quite possible, she told me, for a group of doctors to make nothing at all.

Doctors quickly learn that how much they make has little to do with how good they are. It largely depends on how they handle the business side of their practice. Many doctors expect patients to deal with insurance problems. But that's a recipe for not getting paid. If the doctor sends in a bill and the insurer rejects payment, unless the matter is resolved within ninety days, insurers will pay nothing. Pass the bill on to the patient and many will not pay either. So, to be successful, she said, you have to take on many of the insurance troubles yourself.

"A patient calls to schedule an appointment, and right there things can fall apart," she said. If patients don't have insurance, you have to see if they qualify for a state assistance program like Medicaid. If they do have insurance, you have to find out whether the insurer lists you as a valid physician. You have to make sure the insurer covers the service the patient is seeing you for and find out the stipulations that are made on that service. You have to make sure the patient has the appropriate referral number from his or her primary care physician. You also have to find out if the patient has any copayments or outstanding deductibles to pay, because if so, patients are supposed to bring the money when they see you.

"Patients find this extremely upsetting," Parillo said. "'I have insurance! Why do I have to pay for anything! I didn't bring any money!' Suddenly, you have to be a financial counselor. At the same time, you feel terrible telling them not to come in unless they bring cash, check, or credit card. So you see them anyway, and now you're going to lose 20 percent [about what a copayment covers], which is more than your margin, right off the bat."

Even if all this gets sorted out, there's a further gauntlet of mind-numbing insurance requirements. If you're a surgeon, you may need to obtain a separate referral number for the office visit and for any operation you perform. You may need a preapproval number, too. Afterward, you have to record on the proper billing forms the referral numbers, the preapproval number, the insurance-plan number, the diagnosis codes, the procedure codes, the visit codes, your tax ID number, and any other information the insurer requires. "If you get anything wrong, no money—rejected," Parillo said. Insurers also have

software programs that are designed to reject certain combi-
nations of diagnosis, procedure, and visit codes. Any rejection,
and the full bill goes to the patient. Calls to the insurer produce automated menus and interminable holds.

Parillo's recommendations are pretty straightforward.
Physicians must computerize their billing systems, she said.
They must carefully review the bills they send out and the payments that insurers send back. They must hire office personnel to deal with the insurance companies. A well-run office
can get the insurer's rejection rate down from 30 percent to,
say, 15 percent. That's how a doctor earns money, she told me.
It's a war with insurance, every step of the way.

WHEN I WAS going through medical training, a discouraging
refrain from older physicians was that they would never have
gone into medicine had they known what they know now. A
great many of them simply seemed unable to sort through the
insurance morass. This was perhaps why a 2004 survey of
Massachusetts physicians found that 58 percent were dissatis-
fied with the trade-off between their income and the number
of hours they were working, 56 percent thought their income
was not competitive with what others earn in comparable professions, and 40 percent expected to see their income fall over
the next five years.

William Weeks, a Dartmouth professor, has done a number of studies on the work life of physicians. He and his colleagues found that working hours for physicians are indeed
longer than for other professions. (The typical general surgeon
works sixty-three hours per week.) He also found that, if you

view the expense of going to college and professional school as an investment, the payoff is somewhat poorer in medicine than in some other professions. Tracking the fortunes of graduates of medical schools, law schools, and business schools with comparable entering grade-point averages, he calculated that the annual rate of return by the time they reach middle age is 16 percent per year in primary care medicine, 18 percent in surgery, 23 percent in law, and 26 percent in business. Not bad on the whole, but the differences are there. A physician's income also tends to peak when he or she has been in practice five to ten years and then to decrease in subsequent years as his or her willingness and ability to work the long hours wane.

Yet it seems churlish to complain. Here are the facts. In 2003, the median income for primary care physicians was $156,902. For general surgeons, like me, it was $264,375. In certain specialties, the income can be a good deal higher. Busy orthopedic surgeons, cardiologists, pain specialists, oncologists, neurosurgeons, hand surgeons, and radiologists frequently earn more than half a million dollars a year. Maybe lawyers and businessmen can do better. But then most biochemists, architects, math professors earn less. In the end, are we working for the profits or for the patients? We can count ourselves lucky that we don't have to choose.

There are, however, those who do choose—and manage to earn considerably more than most. I talked to one such surgeon. He had practiced general surgery at the same East Coast hospital for three decades. He loved his work, he said. He did not have an unduly heavy schedule. His office hours were from nine thirty to three thirty on just one day a week. He did about six operations a week. He had been able to develop a

special interest and skill in laparoscopy—performing operations through tiny incisions using fine instruments and a fiber-
optic video camera. And he no longer had to cover midnight
emergencies. I asked him in some roundabout way how much
he earned doing this. "Net income?" he said. "About one point
two million last year."

I had to catch my breath for a moment. He'd made more
than a million dollars every year for at least the past decade. I
wondered how it was possible, or acceptable, to earn so much
for doing general surgery. He was perfectly aware of the reaction. (As was his hospital, which did not want his or its name
to appear in print on the subject.) "I think doctors shortchange
themselves," he said. "Doctors are working for fees that are
similar to or below those of plumbers or electricians"—people
who, he noted, don't require a decade of school and training.
He doesn't see why doctors should let insurance companies
dictate their compensation. So he accepts no insurance. If you
decide to see him, you pay cash. If you then want to fight with
your insurer for reimbursement, that's up to you.

The fees he charges are what he finds the market will
bear. For a laparoscopic cholecystectomy—removal of the
gallbladder, one of the most common operations in general
surgery—insurers will pay surgeons about seven hundred dollars. He asks for eighty-five hundred dollars. For a gastric fun-
doplication, an operation to stop severe reflux of stomach
acid, insurers pay eleven hundred dollars. He charges twelve
thousand dollars. He has had no shortage of patients.

It's not clear how easily others would replicate his success.
After all, he works in a large metropolis, where many people
have either incomes or insurance policies generous enough to

accommodate his fees. He's also something of a star in his field. "I know in my heart that I can do things that other surgeons can't," he told me.

But suppose I did what he did—refused to deal with insurance and charged what the market would bear. I would not make millions, but I could make a lot more than I otherwise would. I'd avoid all the insurance hassles, too. Still, would I want to be a doctor only to those who could afford me?

Why not? the surgeon was asking. "For doctors to think we have to be altruistic is sticking our heads in the sand," he told me. Everyone is squeezing us in order to make money, he said—everyone from the supply companies that we pay to the insurers who are supposed to pay us. In 2005, "the CEO of Aetna's compensation [was] ten million dollars," he pointed out. "These are for-profit companies. Insurance companies make money by withholding reimbursements to physicians or by not approving payment for a service we've provided." To him, the question is why we deal with them at all. In his view, doctors need to understand that we are businessmen—nothing less, nothing more—and the sooner we accept this the better.

His position has a certain bracing clarity. Yet, if this is purely a service-for-money business, if doctoring is no different from selling cars, why choose to endure twelve years of medical training, instead of, say, two years of business school? The reason has to be that doctors remain at least partly motivated by the hope of doing meaningful and respected work for people and society. Thus the responsibility most of us feel to take care of people even when their insurers exasperate us or when they have no insurance at all. If we fail ordinary people, then the notion that we do something special is gone. I can understand wanting to escape the insurance morass. But isn't there some other way around it?

In 1971, a thirty-three-year-old internist named Harris Berman decided to do things a little differently. He and a friend who had just completed his general-surgery training moved back to their home state of New Hampshire, to the town of Nashua. They joined up with a pediatrician, a family practitioner, and an obstetrician. Together they offered health care to patients for a fixed annual fee, without any bills to insurance companies. It was a radical experiment. They paid themselves fixed salaries of thirty thousand dollars a year, a modest income for a doctor at the time, with no differences between specialties. They also bought reinsurance coverage to pay for costs that exceeded fifty thousand dollars, as Berman remembers it, in case a patient developed a catastrophic illness.

The scheme worked. Berman, who is now sixty-eight years old, told me the tale. They called themselves the Matthew Thornton Health Plan, after a physician who was one of New Hampshire's three signers of the Declaration of Independence. They were essentially an HMO, though a very tiny one. Within a short time, about five thousand patients had signed up. The doctors thrived, and there were remarkably few hassles. In the beginning, they didn't have any sub-specialists, so when patients were sent to an ophthalmologist or an orthopedist the Thornton doctors had to pay for the visits. Eventually, they asked the specialists to accept a flat fee each month and dispense with the paperwork.

"Some accepted," Berman said. "And the effect on care

was remarkable. The urologists, for example, suddenly became interested in having us understand which patients they really needed to see and which ones we could take care of without them. They came down and gave us talks—how to work up patients with blood in the urine and decide which ones you had to worry about. The ophthalmologists came down and told us how to take care of itchy eyes and runny eyes. They weren't going to make more money seeing these unnecessary patients, and they found a way to make sure we became more efficient."

After a few years, the Matthew Thornton Health Plan started to be cheaper than other insurers. Employers caught on and enrollment soared. Berman had to bring in more doctors. That's when things got more complicated. "In the beginning, we were all committed," he said. "We worked hard—long hours, a lot of dedication, young and hungry. Then, as we started to get bigger and bring in more staff, we found that others joined for other reasons. They liked the salaried lifestyle—the idea that being a doc could be a job rather than a day-and-night commitment. Some were part-timers. We began to see people looking at their watches as five o'clock approached. It became clear that we had a productivity problem." Also, when they tried to bring in specialists to work full-time with the group, the specialists refused to accept the same salary as the others. In order to get an orthopedic surgeon to join, Berman had to pay him considerably more than what everyone else got. It was the first of many adjustments he had to make in how and what to pay his fellow physicians.

Over the course of thirty years, Berman told me, he ended up trying to pay physicians in almost every conceivable way. He'd paid low salaries and high salaries and still watched them go home at three in the afternoon. He'd paid fee-for-service and watched the paperwork accumulate and the doctors run up the bills to make more money. He'd come up with complicated bonus schemes for productivity and given doctors budgets to oversee. He'd given patients cash accounts to pay their doctors themselves. But no system was able to provide both simplicity and the right balance of thriftiness and reward for good patient care.

By the mid-1980s, sixty thousand patients had joined the Matthew Thornton Health Plan, mainly because it had controlled its costs more successfully than other plans. It had become the second-largest insurer in New Hampshire. And now it was Berman and his rules and his contracts that the physicians complained about. In 1986, Berman left Matthew Thornton, and it was later taken over by Blue Cross. He went on to become the chief executive officer of Tufts Health Plan, one of New England's largest health insurers (where he earned a CEO's income himself). The radical experiment was over.

IN 2005, the United States spent more than two trillion dollars—one-sixth of all the money we have—on health care. This amounted to $7,110 per person. Government and private insurance split about 80 percent of those costs, and the rest largely came out of patients' pockets. Hospitals took about a third of the money; clinicians took another third; and the rest went for other things—nursing homes, prescription drugs, and the costs of administering our insurance system. Americans seem to be reasonably happy with their care, but they haven't liked the prices—insurance premiums increased by 9.2 percent in 2005.

Physicians' after-expense incomes are a fairly small percentage of medical costs. But we're responsible for most of the spending. For the patients I see in the office in a single day, I prescribe somewhere around thirty thousand dollars' worth of medical care—in the form of specialist consultations, surgical procedures, hospital stays, X-ray imaging, and medicines. And how well these services are reimbursed inevitably affects how lavish I can be in dispensing them. This is where money-mindedness becomes inescapable—and likewise the struggle between doing right and doing well.

I remember, twelve years ago, getting the bill for the heart surgery that saved my son Walker's life. The total cost, it said, was almost a quarter-million dollars. My payment? Five dollars—the cost of the copay for the initial visit to the emergency room and the doctor who figured out that our pale and struggling boy was suffering from heart failure. I was an intern then and in no position to pay for any significant part of his medical expenses. If my wife and I had had to, we would have bankrupted ourselves for him. But insurance meant that all anyone—either us or his doctors and nurses—had to consider was his needs. It was a beautiful thing. Yet it's also the source of what economists call "moral hazard": with other people paying the bills, I did not care how much was spent or charged to save my child. To me, all the members of the team deserved a million dollars for what they did. Others were footing the bill—so it's left to them to question the price. Hence the adversarial relationship patients and doctors have with insurers. Whether insurance is provided by the government or by corporations, there is no reason to think that the battles—over the fees charged, the bills rejected, the preapproval contortions—will ever end.

Given the struggles over payment, what's striking is how substantial medical reimbursements have continued to be. Physicians in the United States today remain better compensated than physicians anywhere else in the world. Our earnings are more than seven times those of the average American employee, and that gap has grown over time. (In most industrialized countries, the ratio is under three.) This has allowed American medicine to attract enormous talent to its ranks and kept doctors willing to work harder than members of almost any other profession. At the same time, we as a country have shown little concern for the uninsured. One American in seven has no coverage, and one in three younger than sixty-five will lose coverage at some point in the next two years. These are people who aren't poor or old enough to qualify for government programs but whose jobs aren't good enough to provide benefits, either. They face difficulty finding doctors who will treat them, unconscionable rates of bankruptcy from health care bills, and a proven increased likelihood that problems such as high blood pressure, heart disease, appendicitis, and cancer will go undetected or inadequately treated. Our byzantine insurance system leaves gaps at every turn. Some day soon that must change.

A FEW DAYS after the chairman of surgery offered me the job, I returned to his office and named my figure.

"That'll do fine," he said, and we shook hands. Now I am the one who's too embarrassed to say what I earn. We talked for a while afterward: about how to fit research in, about how many nights I'd have to be on call, about how to keep time for my family. The prospect of my new responsibilities filled me with both exhilaration and dread.

As the meeting was ending, though, I realized that there was one final important question I had not brought up.

"What are the health insurance benefits like?" I asked.

The Doctors of the Death Chamber

O n February 14, 2006, a United States district court issued an unprecedented ruling concerning the California execution by lethal injection of murderer Michael Morales. The ruling ordered the state to have a physician, specifically an anesthesiologist, personally supervise the execution or else to drastically change the standard protocol for lethal injections. Under that protocol, the anesthetic sodium thiopental is given at massive doses that are expected to halt breathing and extinguish consciousness within one minute after administration; then the paralytic agent pancuronium is given, followed by a fatal dose of potassium chloride. The judge found, however, that evidence from execution logs showed that six of the previous eight prisoners put to death in

California had not stopped breathing before technicians gave the paralytic agent; the finding raised a serious possibility that the prisoners had experienced suffocation from the paralytic, a feeling much like being buried alive, and felt intense pain from the potassium bolus. This experience would be unacceptable under the Constitution's Eighth Amendment protections against cruel and unusual punishment. So the judge ordered the state to have an anesthesiologist present in the death chamber to determine when the prisoner was unconscious enough for the second and third injections to be given—or to have a general physician supervise an execution performed with sodium thiopental alone.

The California Medical Association, the American Medical Association (AMA), and the American Society of Anesthesiologists (ASA) immediately and loudly opposed such physician participation as a clear violation of medical ethics codes. "Physicians are healers, not executioners," the ASA's president told reporters. Nonetheless, in just two days, prison officials announced that they had found two willing anesthesiologists. The court agreed to maintain their anonymity and to allow them to shield their identities from witnesses. Both withdrew the day before the execution, however, after the Court of Appeals for the Ninth Circuit added a further stipulation requiring them to personally administer additional medication if the prisoner remained conscious or exhibited pain. This they would not accept. The execution was then postponed (Morales remained on death row as of January 2007), but federal courts have since continued to require that medical professionals assist with the administration of any execution by lethal injection.

Execution has become a medical procedure in the United States. That fact has forced a few doctors and nurses, asked to participate in executions, to choose between the ethical codes of their professions and the desires of broader society. The codes of medical societies are not always right and neither are the laws of society. There are vital but sometimes murky differences between acting skillfully, acting lawfully, and acting ethically. So how individual doctors and nurses have sorted these out and made their choices interested me.

The *Morales* ruling is the culmination of a steady evolution in methods of execution in the United States. On July 2, 1976, in deciding the case of *Gregg v. Georgia,* the Supreme Court legalized capital punishment after a decadelong moratorium on executions. Executions resumed six months later, on January 17, 1977, in Utah, with the death by firing squad of Gary Gilmore for the killing of Ben Bushnell, a Provo motel manager.

Death by firing squad, however, came to be regarded as too bloody and uncontrolled. (Gilmore's heart, for example, did not stop until two minutes after he was shot, and shooters have sometimes weakened at the trigger, as famously happened in 1951 in Utah when the five riflemen fired away from the target over Elisio Mares's heart, only to hit his right chest and cause him to bleed slowly to death.)

Hanging came to be regarded as still more inhumane. Under the best of circumstances, the cervical spine is broken at the second vertebra, the diaphragm is paralyzed, and the prisoner suffocates to death, a minutes-long process.

Gas chambers proved no better: asphyxiation from cyanide gas, which prevents cells from using oxygen by inactivating a vital enzyme known as cytochrome oxidase, took even longer than death by hanging, and the public revolted at the vision of suffocating prisoners fighting for air and then seizing as their ability to use oxygen shut down. In Arizona, in 1992, for example, the asphyxiation of triple murderer Donald Harding took eleven minutes, and the sight was so horrifying that reporters cried, the attorney general vomited, and the prison warden announced he would resign if forced to conduct another such execution. Since 1976, only two prisoners have been executed by firing squad, three by hanging, and eleven by gas chamber.

Many more executions, 74 of the first hundred after *Gregg* and 153 in all, were by electrocution, which was thought to cause a swifter, more acceptable death. But officials found that the electrical flow frequently arced, cooking flesh and sometimes igniting prisoners—postmortem examinations often had to be delayed for the bodies to cool—and yet in the case of some prisoners, it took repeated jolts to kill them. In Alabama, in 1979, for example, John Louis Evans III was still alive after two cycles of 2,600 volts; the warden called Governor George Wallace, who told him to keep going, and only after a third cycle, with witnesses screaming in the gallery, and almost twenty minutes of suffering, did Evans finally die. Only Florida, Virginia, and Alabama persisted with electrocutions with any frequency, and under threat of Supreme Court review, they too abandoned the method.

Lethal injection now appears to be the sole method of execution accepted by courts as humane enough to satisfy Eighth Amendment requirements—largely because it medicalizes the process. The prisoner is laid supine on a hospital gurney. A white bedsheet is drawn to his chest. An intravenous line flows into his arm. Under the protocol devised in 1977 by Dr. Stanley Deutsch, the chairman of anesthesiology at the University of Oklahoma, prisoners are first given 2,500 to 5,000 milligrams of sodium thiopental (five to ten times the recommended maximum for ordinary therapeutic use), which can produce death all by itself by causing complete cessation of the brain's electrical activity, followed by respiratory arrest and circulatory collapse. Death, however, can take fifteen minutes or longer with thiopental alone, and the prisoner may appear to gasp, struggle, or convulse. So 60 to 100 milligrams of pancuronium (ten times the usual dose) is injected one minute or so after the thiopental to paralyze the prisoner's muscles. Finally, 120 to 240 milliequivalents of potassium is given to produce rapid cardiac arrest.

Officials liked this method. Because it borrowed from established anesthesia techniques, it made execution more like familiar medical procedures than the grisly, backlash-inducing spectacle it had become. (In Missouri, executions were even moved to a prison-hospital procedure room.) It was less disturbing to witness. The drugs were cheap and routinely available. (Cyanide gas and 30,000-watt electrical generators, by comparison, were awfully hard to find.) And officials could turn to doctors and nurses to help with technical difficulties, attest to the painlessness and trustworthiness of the technique, and lend a more professional air to the proceedings.

But medicine balked. In 1980, when the first execution was planned using Deutsch's technique, the AMA passed a resolution against physician participation as a violation of core medical ethics. The resolution was quite general. It did not address, for example, whether pronouncing death at the scene—something doctors had done at previous executions—was acceptable or not. So the AMA clarified the ban in its 1992 Code of Medical Ethics. Article 2.06 states, "A physician, as a member of a profession dedicated to preserving life when there is hope of doing so, should not be a participant in a legally authorized execution," although an individual physician's opinion about capital punishment remains "the personal moral decision of the individual." The code further stipulates that unacceptable participation includes prescribing or administering medications as part of the execution procedure, monitoring vital signs, rendering technical advice, selecting injection sites, starting or supervising placement of intravenous lines, or simply being present as a physician. Pronouncing death is also considered unacceptable, because the physician is not permitted to revive the prisoner if he or she is found to be alive. Only two actions are acceptable: provision, at the prisoner's request, of a sedative to calm anxiety beforehand and signing a death certificate after another person has pronounced death.

The code of ethics of the Society of Correctional Physicians establishes an even stricter ban: "The correctional health professional shall . . . not be involved in any aspect of execution of the death penalty." The American Nurses Association (ANA) has adopted a similar prohibition. Only the national pharmacists' society, the American Pharmaceutical Association, permits involvement, accepting the voluntary provision of execution medications by pharmacists as ethical conduct.

States, however, wanted a medical presence. In 1982, in Texas, the state prison medical director, Ralph Gray, and another doctor, Bascom Bentley, agreed to attend the country's first execution by lethal injection, though only to pronounce death. But once on the scene, Gray was persuaded to examine the prisoner to show the team the best injection site. Still, the doctors refused to give advice about the injection itself and simply watched as the warden prepared the chemicals. When he tried to push the syringe, however, it did not work. He had mixed all the drugs together, and they had precipitated into a clot of white sludge.

"I could have told you that," one of the doctors reportedly said, shaking his head.

After a second effort, Gray went to pronounce the prisoner dead but found him still alive. The doctors were part of the team now, though; they suggested allowing time for more drugs to run in.

Today, all thirty-eight death-penalty states rely on lethal injection. Of 1,045 murderers executed since 1976, 876 were executed by injection. Against vigorous opposition from the AMA and state medical societies, thirty-five of the thirty-eight states explicitly allow physician participation in executions. Indeed, seventeen require it: Colorado, Florida, Georgia, Idaho, Louisiana, Mississippi, Nevada, North Carolina, New Hampshire, New Jersey, New Mexico, Oklahoma, Oregon, South Dakota, Virginia, Washington, and Wyoming. To protect participating physicians from license challenges for violating ethics codes, states commonly promise anonymity and provide legal immunity from such challenges. Nonetheless, despite the promised anonymity, several states have produced the physicians in court to vouch publicly for the legitimacy and painlessness of the procedure. And despite the immunity, several physicians have faced license challenges, though none have lost as yet.

States have affirmed that physicians and nurses—including those who are prison employees—have a right to refuse to participate in any way in executions. Yet they have found physicians and nurses who are willing to participate. Who are these people? Why do they do it?

IT IS NOT easy to find answers to these questions. Medical personnel who help with executions are difficult to identify and reluctant to discuss their roles, even when offered anonymity. Among the fifteen I was able to locate, however, I found four physicians and one nurse who agreed to speak with me; collectively, they have helped with at least forty-five executions. None were zealots for the death penalty, and none had a simple explanation for why they did this work. The role, most said, had crept up on them.

Dr. A has helped with about eight executions in his state. He was extremely uncomfortable talking about the subject. Nonetheless, he ultimately agreed to tell me his story.

Almost sixty years old, he is board certified in internal medicine and critical care, and he and his family have lived in their small town for thirty years. He is well respected. Almost everyone of local standing comes to see him as their primary care physician—the bankers, his fellow doctors, the mayor. Among his patients is the warden of the maximum-security prison that happens to be in his town. One day several years ago, the two of them got talking during an appointment. The warden complained of difficulties staffing the prison clinic and asked Dr. A if he would be willing to see prisoners there occasionally. Dr. A said he would. He'd have made more money in his own clinic—the prison paid sixty-five dollars an hour—but the prison was important to the community, he liked the warden, and it was just a few hours of work a month. He was happy to help.

Then, a year or two later, the warden asked him for help with a different problem. The state had a death penalty, and the legislature had voted to use lethal injection exclusively. The executions were to be carried out in the warden's prison. He needed doctors, he said. Would Dr. A help? He would not have to deliver the lethal injection. He would just help with cardiac monitoring. The warden gave the doctor time to consider the request.

"My wife didn't like it," Dr. A told me. "She said, 'Why do you want to go there?'" But he felt torn. "I knew something about the past of these killers." One of them had killed a mother of three during a convenience-store robbery and then, while getting away, shot a man who was standing at his car. Another convict had kidnapped, raped, and strangled to death an eleven-year-old girl. "I do not have a very strong conviction about the death penalty, but I don't feel anything negative about it for such people either. The execution order was given legally by the court. And morally, if you think about the animal behavior of some of these people. . . ." Ultimately, he decided to participate, he said, because he was only helping with monitoring, because he was needed by the warden and his community, because the sentence was society's order, and because the punishment did not seem wrong.

At the first execution, he was instructed to stand behind a curtain watching the inmate's heart rhythm on a cardiac monitor. Neither the witnesses on the other side of a glass window nor the prisoner could see him. A technician placed two IV lines. Someone he could not see pushed the three drugs, one right after another. Watching the monitor, he saw the normal rhythm slow, then the waveforms widen. He recognized the tall peaks of potassium toxicity, followed by the fine spikes of ventricular fibrillation, and finally the flat, unwavering line of an asystolic cardiac arrest. He waited half a minute, then signaled to another physician, who went out before the witnesses to place his stethoscope on the prisoner's unmoving chest. The doctor listened for thirty seconds and then told the warden the inmate was dead. Half an hour later, Dr. A was released. He made his way through a side door, past the crowd gathered outside, to his parked car and headed home.

In three subsequent executions there were difficulties, though, all with finding a vein for an IV. The prisoners were either obese or past intravenous drug users, or both. The technicians would stick and stick and, after half an hour, give up. This was a possibility the warden had not prepared for. Dr. A had placed numerous lines. Could he give a try?

OK, Dr. A decided. Let me take a look.

This was a turning point, though he didn't recognize it at the time. He was there to help, they had a problem, and so he would help. It did not occur to him to do otherwise.

In two of the prisoners, he told me, he found a good vein and placed the IV. In one, however, he could not find a vein. All eyes were on him. He felt responsible for the situation. The prisoner was calm. Dr. A remembered the prisoner saying to him, almost to comfort him, "No, they can never get the vein." The doctor decided to place a central line, an intravenous line that goes directly into the chest. People scrambled to find a kit.

I asked him how he placed the line. It was like placing one "for any other patient," he said. He decided to place it in the subclavian vein, a thick pipe of a vein running under the collarbone, because that is what he most commonly did. He opened the kit for the triple-lumen catheter and explained to the prisoner everything he was going to do. I asked him if he was afraid of the prisoner. "No," he said. The man was perfectly cooperative. Dr. A put on sterile gloves, gown, and mask. He swabbed the man's skin with antiseptic.

"Why?" I asked.

"Habit," he said. He injected a local anesthetic. He punctured the vein with one stick. He checked to make sure he had a good, nonpulsatile flow of dark venous blood coming out. He threaded a guide wire through the needle, a dilator over the guide wire, and finally slid the catheter in. All went smoothly. He flushed the lines with saline, secured the catheter to the skin with a stitch, and put a clean dressing on, just as he always does. Then he went back behind the curtain to monitor the lethal injection.

Only one case seemed to really bother him. The convict, who had killed a policeman, weighed about 350 pounds. The team placed his intravenous lines without trouble. But after they had given him all three injections, the prisoner's heart rhythm continued. "It was an agonal rhythm," Dr. A said, a rhythm with a widened appearance on the EKG, going only ten or twenty beats per minute. "He was dead," he insisted.

Nonetheless, the rhythm continued. The team looked to Dr. A. His explanation of what happened next diverges from what I learned from another source. I was told that he instructed that another bolus of potassium be given. When I asked him if he did, he said, "No, I didn't. As far as I remember, I didn't say anything. I think it may have been another physician." Certainly, however, all boundary lines had been crossed. He had agreed to take part in the executions simply to watch a cardiac monitor, but just by being present, by having expertise, he had opened himself to being called on to do steadily more, to take responsibility for the execution itself. Perhaps he was not the executioner. But he was darn close to it. And he seemed troubled by that.

I asked him whether he had known that his actions—everything from his monitoring the executions to helping officials with the process of delivering the drugs—violated the AMA's ethics code. "I never had any inkling," he said. And indeed, the only survey done on this issue, in 1999, found that just 3 percent of doctors knew of any guidelines governing their participation in executions. The humaneness of a lethal injection Dr. A was involved in was challenged in court, however. The state summoned him for a public deposition on the process, including the particulars of the execution in which the prisoner required a central line. His local newspaper printed the story. Word spread through his town. Not long after, he arrived at work to find a sign pasted to his clinic door reading, THE KILLER DOCTOR. A challenge to his medical license was filed with the state. If he wasn't aware earlier that there was an ethical issue at stake, he was now.

Ninety percent of his patients supported him, he said,

and the state medical board upheld his license under a law that defined participation in executions as acceptable activity for a physician. But he decided that he wanted no part of the controversy anymore and quit. He still defends what he did. Had he known of the AMA's position, though, "I never would have gotten involved," he said.

DR. B SPOKE to me between clinic appointments. He is a family physician, and he has participated in some thirty executions. He became involved long ago, when electrocution was the primary method, and then continued through the transition to lethal injections. He remains a participant to this day. But it was apparent that he had been more cautious and reflective about his involvement than Dr. A had. He also seemed more troubled by it.

Dr. B, too, had first been approached by a patient. "One of my patients was a prison investigator," he said. "I never quite understood his role, but he was an intermediary between the state and the inmates. He was hired to monitor that the state was taking care of them. They had the first two executions after the death penalty was reinstated, and there was a problem with the second one, where the physicians were going in a minute or so after the event and still hearing heartbeats. The two physicians were doing this out of courtesy, because the facility was in their area. But the case unnerved them to the point that they quit. The officials had a lot of trouble finding another doctor after that. So that was when my patient talked to me."

Dr. B did not really want to get involved. He was in his

forties then. He'd gone to a top-tier medical school. He'd protested the Vietnam War in the 1960s. "I've gone from a radical hippie to a middle-class American over the years," he said. "I wasn't on any bandwagons anymore." But his patient said the team needed a physician only to pronounce death. Dr. B had no personal objection to capital punishment. So in the moment—"it was a quick judgment"—he agreed, "but only to do the pronouncement."

The execution was a few days later by electric chair. It was an awful sight, he said. "They say an electrocution is not an issue. But when someone comes up out of that chair six inches, it's not for nothing." He waited a long while before going out to the prisoner. When he did, he performed a systematic examination. He checked for a carotid pulse. He listened to the man's heart three times with a stethoscope. He looked for a pupil response with his penlight. Only then did he pronounce the man dead.

He thought harder about whether to stay involved after that first time. "I went to the library and researched it," and that was when he discovered the 1980 AMA guidelines. As he understood the code, if he did nothing except make a pronouncement of death, he would be acting properly and ethically. (This was before the 1992 AMA clarification that made pronouncing death at the scene a clear violation of the code, but allowed signing a death certificate afterward.)

Knowing the guidelines reassured him about his involvement and made him willing to continue. It also emboldened him to draw thicker boundaries around his participation. During the first lethal injections, he and another physician "were in the room when they were administering the drugs," he said.

"We could see the telemetry [the cardiac monitor]. We could see a lot of things. But I had them remove us from that area. I said, 'I do not want any access to the monitor or the EKGs.' . . . A couple times they asked me about recommendations in cases in which there were venous access problems. I said, 'No. I'm not going to assist in any way.' They would ask about amounts of medicines. They had problems getting the medicines. But I said I had no interest in getting involved in any of that."

Dr. B kept himself at some remove from the execution process, but he would be the first to admit that his is not an ethically pristine position. When he refused to provide additional assistance, the execution team simply found others who would. He was glad to have those people there. "If the doctors and nurses are removed, I don't think [lethal injections] could be competently or predictably done. I can tell you I wouldn't be involved unless those people were involved.

"I agonize over the ethics of this every time they call me to go down there," he said. His wife knew about his involvement from early on, but he could not bring himself to tell his children until they were grown. He has let almost no one else know. Even his medical staff is unaware.

The trouble is not that the lethal injections seem cruel to him. "Mostly, they are very peaceful," he said. The agonizing comes instead from his doubts about whether anything is accomplished. "The whole system doesn't seem right," he told me toward the end of our conversation. "I guess I see more and more executions, and I really wonder. . . . It just seems like the justice system is going down a dead-end street. I can't say that [lethal injection] lessens the incidence of anything.

The real depressing thing is that if you don't get to these people before the age of three or four or five, it's not going to make any difference in what they do. They've struck out before they even started kindergarten. I don't see [executions] as saying anything about that."

THE MEDICAL PEOPLE most wary of speaking to me were those who worked as full-time employees in state prison systems. Nonetheless, two did agree to speak, one a physician in a southern state prison and the other a nurse who had worked in a prison out west. Both seemed less conflicted about being involved in executions than Dr. A or Dr. B.

The physician, Dr. C, was younger than the others and relatively junior among his prison's doctors. He did not trust me to keep his identity confidential, and I think he worried for his job if anyone found out about our conversation. As a result, although I had independent information that he had participated in at least two executions, he would speak only in general terms about the involvement of doctors. But he was clear about what he believed.

"I think that if you're going to work in the correctional setting, [participating in executions] is potentially a component of what you need to do," he said. "It is only a tiny part of anything that you're doing as part of your public health service. A lot of society thinks these people should not get any care at all." But in his job he must follow the law and it obligates him to provide proper care, he said. It also has set the prisoners' punishment. "Thirteen jurors, citizens of the state, have made a decision. And if I live in that state and that's the law, then I would see it as being an obligation to be available."

He explained further. "I think that if I had to face someone I loved being put to death, I would want that done by lethal injection, and I would want to know that it is done competently."

The nurse saw his participation in fairly similar terms. He had fought as a marine in Vietnam and later became a nurse. As an army reservist, he served with a surgical unit in Bosnia and in Iraq. He worked for many years on critical care units and, for almost a decade, as nurse manager for a busy emergency department. He then took a job as the nurse in charge for his state penitentiary, where he helped with one execution by lethal injection.

It was the state's first execution by this method, and "at the time, there was great naïveté about lethal injection," he said. "No one in that state had any idea what was involved." The warden had a protocol from Texas and thought it looked pretty simple. What did he need medical personnel for? The warden told the nurse that he would start the IVs himself, though he had never started one before.

"Are you, as a doctor, going to let this person stab the inmate for half an hour because of his inexperience?" the nurse asked me. "I wasn't." He said, "I had no qualms. If this is to be done correctly, if it is to be done at all, then I am the person to do it."

This is not to say that he felt easy about it, however. "As a marine and as a nurse, . . . I hope I will never become someone who has no problem taking another person's life." But society had decided the punishment and had done so carefully with multiple judicial reviews, he said. The convict had killed four people even while in prison. He had arranged for an accomplice to blow up the home of a county attorney he was angry with while the attorney, his wife, and their child were inside. When the accomplice turned state's evidence, the inmate arranged for him to be tortured and killed at a roadside rest stop. The nurse did not disagree with the final judgment that this man should be put to death.

The nurse took his involvement seriously. "As the leader of the health care team," he said, "it was my responsibility to make sure that everything be done in a way that was professional and respectful to the inmate as a human being." He spoke to an official with the state nursing board about the process, and although involvement is against the ANA's ethics code, the board said that under state law he was permitted to do everything except push the drugs.

So he issued the purchase request to the pharmacist supplying the drugs. He did a dry run with the public citizen chosen to push the injections and with the guards to make sure they knew how to bring the prisoner out and strap him down. On the day of the execution, the nurse dressed as if for an operation, in scrubs, mask, hat, and sterile gown and gloves. He explained to the prisoner exactly what was going to happen. He placed two IVs and taped them down. The warden read the final order to the prisoner and allowed him his last words. "He didn't say anything about his guilt or his innocence," the nurse said. "He just said that the execution made all of us involved killers just like him."

The warden gave the signal to start the injection. The nurse hooked the syringe to the IV port and told the citizen to push the sodium thiopental. "The inmate started to say, 'Yeah, I can feel . . .' and then he passed out." They completed the injections and, three minutes later, he flatlined on the cardiac monitor. The two physicians on the scene had been left nothing to do except pronounce the inmate dead.

I HAVE PERSONALLY been in favor of the death penalty. I was a senior official in the 1992 Clinton presidential campaign and in the administration, and in that role I defended the president's stance in support of capital punishment. I have no illusions that the death penalty deters anyone from murder. I also have great concern about the ability of our justice system to avoid putting someone innocent to death. However, I believe there are some human beings who do such evil as to deserve to die. I am not troubled that Timothy McVeigh was executed for the 168 people he killed in the Oklahoma City bombing or that John Wayne Gacy was for committing thirty-three murders.

Still, I hadn't thought much about exactly how the executions are done. And I have always instinctively regarded involvement in executions by physicians and nurses as wrong. The public has granted us extraordinary and exclusive dispensation to administer drugs to people, even to the point of unconsciousness, to cut them open, to do what would otherwise be considered assault, because we do so on their behalf—to save their lives and provide them comfort. To have the state take control of these skills for its purposes against a human being—for punishment—seems a dangerous perversion. Society has trusted us with powerful abilities, and the more willing we are to use these abilities against individual people, the more we risk and betray that trust.

My conversations with the physicians and the nurse I had tracked down, however, rattled both these views—and no conversation more so than one I had with the final doctor I spoke to. Dr. D is a forty-five-year-old emergency physician. He is also a volunteer medical director for a shelter for abused children. He works to reduce homelessness. He opposes the death penalty because he regards it as inhumane, immoral, and pointless. And he has participated in six executions so far.

About a decade ago, a new jail was built down the street from the hospital where he worked, and it had a large infirmary "the size of our whole emergency room." The jail needed a doctor. So, out of curiosity as much as anything, Dr. D began working there. "I found that I loved it," he said. "Jails are an underserved niche of health care." Jails, he pointed out, are different from prisons in that they house people who are arrested and awaiting trial. Most are housed only a few hours to days and then released. "The substance abuse and noncompliance is high. The people have a wide variety of medical needs. It is a fascinating population. The setting is very similar to the ER. You can make a tremendous impact on people and on public health." Over time, he shifted more and more of his work to the jail system. He built a medical group for the jails in his area and soon became an advocate for correctional medicine.

In 2002, the doctors who had been involved in executions in his state pulled out. Officials asked Dr. D if his group would take the contract. Before answering, he went to observe an execution. "It was a very emotional experience for

me," he said. "I was shocked to witness something like this."
He had opposed the death penalty since college, and nothing
he saw made him feel any differently. But, at the same time, he
felt there were needs that he as a correctional physician could
serve.

He read about the ethics of participating. He knew
about the AMA's stance against it. Yet he also felt an obligation
not to abandon inmates in their dying moments. "We, as doctors, are not the ones deciding the fate of this individual," he
said. "The way I saw it, this is an end-of-life issue, just as with
any other terminal disease. It just happens that it involves a legal process instead of a medical process. When we have a patient who can no longer survive his illness, we as physicians
must ensure he has comfort. [A death-penalty] patient is no
different from a patient dying of cancer—except his cancer is a
court order." Dr. D said he has "the cure for this cancer"—
abolition of the death penalty—but "if the people and the government won't let you provide it, and a patient then dies, are
you not going to comfort him?"

His group took the contract, and he has been part of the
medical team for each execution since. The doctors are available to help if there are difficulties with IV access, and Dr. D
considers it their task to ensure that the prisoner is without
pain or suffering through the process. He himself provides the
cardiac monitoring and the final determination of death.
Watching the changes on the two-line electrocardiogram tracing, "I keep having that reflex as an ER doctor, wanting to
treat that rhythm," he said. Aside from that, his main reaction
is to be sad for everyone involved—the prisoner whose life has
led to this, the victims, the prison officials, the doctors. The

team's payment is substantial—eighteen thousand dollars—but he donates his portion to the children's shelter where he volunteers.

Three weeks after speaking to me, he told me to go ahead and use his name. It is Carlo Musso. He helps with executions in Georgia. He didn't want to seem as if he were hiding anything, he said. He didn't want to invite trouble, either. But activists have already challenged his license and his membership in the AMA, and he is resigned to the fight. "It just seems wrong for us to walk away, to abdicate our responsibility to the patients," he said.

THERE IS LITTLE doubt that lethal injection can be painless and peaceful, but as courts have recognized, ensuring that it is requires significant medical assistance and judgment—for placement of intravenous lines, monitoring of consciousness, and adjustments in medication timing and dosage. In recent years, medical societies have persuaded two states, Kentucky and Illinois, to pass laws forbidding physician participation in executions. Nonetheless, officials in each of these states intend to continue to rely on medical supervision, employing nurses and nurse anesthetists instead. How, then, to reconcile the conflict between government efforts to provide a medical presence and our ethical principles forbidding it? Are our ethics what should change?

The doctors' and nurse's arguments for competence and comfort in the execution process certainly have force and they gave me pause. But however much these practitioners may wish to comfort a patient, it ultimately seems clear to me that the inmate is not really their patient. Unlike genuine patients, an inmate has no ability to refuse the physician's "care"—indeed, the inmate and his family are not even permitted to know the physician's identity. And the medical assistance provided primarily serves the government's purposes—not the inmate's needs and interests as a patient. Medicine is being made an instrument of punishment. The hand of comfort that more gently places the IV, more carefully times the bolus of potassium, is also the hand of death. We cannot escape this truth.

This truth is what convinces me that we should stand with the ethics code and legally ban the participation of physicians and nurses in executions. And if it turns out that executions cannot then be performed without, as the courts put it, "unconstitutional pain and cruelty," the death penalty should be abolished.

It is far from clear that a society that punishes its most evil murderers with life imprisonment is worse off than one that punishes them with death. But a society in which the government actively subverts core ethical principles of medical practice is patently worse off for it. The U.S. government has shown willingness to use medical skills against individuals for its own purposes—having medical personnel assist in the interrogation of prisoners, for example, adjust their medical documentation and death certificates, place feeding tubes for force-feeding them, and help with executing them. As our abilities to manipulate the human body advance, government interest in our skills will only increase. Preserving the integrity of medical ethics could not be more important.

The four physicians and the nurse I spoke to all acted against long-standing principles of their professions. Their in-

dividual actions have rendered those principles effectively ir-
relevant; as long as a prison can count on a handful of doctors
and nurses helping with executions, the ethics of the many do
not matter. Yet, it must be said, most of those I interviewed
took their moral duties seriously. It is worth reflecting on this
truth as well.

The easy thing for any doctor or nurse is simply to follow
the written rules. But each of us has a duty not to follow rules
and laws blindly. In medicine, we face conflicts about what the
right and best actions are in all kinds of areas: relief of suffering for the terminally ill, provision of narcotics for patients
with chronic pain, withdrawal of life-sustaining treatment for
the critically ill, abortion, and executions, to name just a few.
All have been the subject of professional rules and government regulation, and at times those rules and regulations have
been and will be wrong. We may then be called on to make a
choice. We must do our best to choose intelligently and wisely.

Sometimes, however, we will be wrong—as I think the
doctors and nurses are who have used their privileged skills to
make possible 876 deaths by lethal injection thus far. We each
should then be prepared to accept the consequences. Above
all, we have to be prepared to recognize when using our abilities skillfully comes into conflict with using them rightly. Assistance with executions is a stark instance. But it is far from
the only one. Indeed, it is not even the most difficult one.

On Fighting

I used to think that the hardest struggle of doctoring is learning the skills. But it is not, although just when you begin to feel confident that you know what you are doing, a failure knocks you down. It is not the strain of the work, either, though sometimes you are worn to your ragged edge. No, the hardest part of being a doctor, I have found, is to know what you have power over and what you don't.

I have a patient, Mr. Thomas, who came to see me in my clinic one autumn with Cushing's syndrome, a hormonal disease in which the adrenal glands become enlarged and start pouring out massive amounts of cortisol, a steroid hormone. It is as if a person is being given a constant intravenous steroid overdose. And these steroids aren't the kind that build up your muscle; they are the kind that break it down.

Thomas is seventy-two. Until that year, he had been a vigorous man enjoying retirement on Cape Cod with his wife after a career teaching high school history in New York City. He'd been healthy. He took medication for blood pressure and an arthritis that intermittently flared in his right hip, and that was all. The previous winter, however, a question on an X-ray led to a CT scan which revealed a three-inch mass, a cancer, in his left kidney. In retrospect, the adrenal glands looked slightly plump on the scan, but not terribly so, and the cancer was the greater concern. Thomas underwent surgery to remove his kidney. The cancer appeared to have been caught in time, and he recovered without difficulties.

Over the next few months, however, Thomas developed marked swelling of his face, his legs, his arms. He looked rounder, even bloated. He began bruising easily. He developed strange, recurrent pneumonias—fungal pneumonias that usually only afflict people on chemotherapy or with HIV. He was a puzzle to his doctors. They carried out all kinds of tests and eventually his sky-high levels of cortisol were found—Cushing's syndrome. Repeat scans showed that his adrenal glands had grown to at least four times normal size and that they were producing the steroid overload. The doctors did more tests to find the cause of the adrenal surge—a pituitary gland malfunction is a common one, for example—but none was found. He became increasingly weak and so tired that just moving required colossal effort. That summer, he began having difficulty climbing stairs. By September, he struggled just to stand from sitting. His endocrinologist tried medications to counteract the hormone. But by November, Thomas couldn't stand at all and was bound to a wheelchair. The pneumonias continued to reappear despite antifungal treatments. The hormones flowing uncontrolled out of his adrenal glands were destroying his muscles and shutting down his immune system.

He was sent to see me for a consultation just before Thanksgiving. His wife could not hide the alarm on her face, but he himself was calm, even commanding, despite his wheelchair and the alien, white fluorescent examination room. He was six foot one, of Afro-Caribbean origin, and when he spoke it was clearly and directly, like a man used to the authority of a classroom. I got straight to the point. I told him the only option that could fix his adrenal problem was to remove both of his adrenal glands. I explained that the glands sit atop the kidneys like two fleshy yellow tricornered hats— the right gland is tucked under the liver, the left behind the stomach—and that removing both is a drastic measure. It replaces the problems of having too much hormone with those of having too little: low blood pressure, depression, yet worse fatigue, and a critical inability to muster a stress response to infection or trauma—though hormone pills generally mitigate these effects. The operation is also a major one, with potential for serious complications ranging from bleeding to organ failure, especially given his declining health and the previous operation he'd had to remove his cancerous kidney. If he didn't go through with it, however, it was clear that he would dwindle away and die in a matter of months.

Thomas did not want to die. But he confessed to being more afraid of the surgery and what it might do to him. He didn't want pain. He didn't want to be away from home. I told him he needed to set his fears aside. I asked him, what were his hopes? He wanted to have a normal life, he said, to be with his wife, to walk the beach near his house again. This was why he should have the operation, I said. No question, there were serious risks. The recovery would be hard. The operation might not work. But it was his only chance, and if all went well, the life he hoped for was possible. He agreed to go ahead.

Technically, the surgery went as smoothly as it could have. With the removal of his adrenal glands, his cortisol level plummeted and could be held in a normal range with medications. He is no longer dying. But seven months after the surgery, as I write this, he has still not gotten home. For three weeks, he was in a coma. His pneumonias recurred. We had to put in a tracheostomy and a feeding tube. Then he developed an abdominal infection that required the insertion of multiple drainage tubes. He developed sepsis from two different bacteria floating around the hospital. He spent a total of four months in intensive care, and the debility only destroyed more of what little muscle he had remaining.

Thomas is now in a long-term care facility. He was brought to my office recently, by ambulance, on a stretcher. He was gaining strength, the rehabilitation doctors told me, but in the office he had difficulty just lifting his head off the pillow. I covered his tracheostomy so he could talk. He asked me when he would be able to stand again, to go home. I didn't know, I told him, and he began to cry.

We have at our disposal today the remarkable abilities of modern medicine. Learning to use them is difficult enough. But understanding their limits is the most difficult task of all.

★   ★   ★

ONE DAY MY wife's New Hampshire cousins called me about their twelve-year-old daughter, Callie. A little over a year earlier, she began to feel unexpectedly short of breath. A chest X-ray showed a mass filling her chest. It was a lymphoma—not unlike the one Peter Franklin had got as a medical student. This one was the non-Hodgkin's type, which doctors can cure in more than 80 percent of children at her stage of disease. Callie was given a standard six-month course of chemotherapy. Her hair fell out. Her mouth blistered. She became weakened and nauseated. But the cancer disappeared. Then, several months later, her tumor was found to have grown back, just as big as before. When a lymphoma returns after chemotherapy, the textbooks do not give statistics. They only say, "The prognosis is poor." Callie's oncologist had treatment options, though. She and the family decided to try a new chemotherapy. But after the initial dose, Callie's white blood cell count dropped alarmingly. It took her weeks in the hospital to recover. Her oncologist discussed further courses of action with Callie and her family. Together they decided to press ahead with yet a different chemotherapy. Again, her white blood cell count fell alarmingly. The tumor did not shrink a centimeter.

That was when her father, Robin, and I spoke. He did not know what to do. The cancer had grown despite three different chemotherapy regimens. Callie had had to have a half-inch-thick tube put into her chest to drain the fluid accumulating from the cancer. She was unbearably nauseated again. Her vomiting made it difficult for her to eat. She was exhausted and emaciated. Between the chest tube, the cancer, the needle sticks, and the bandage changes, she felt pain almost every hour. There were options still left—other chemotherapies, experimental treatments, possibly even bone marrow transplantation. But how real were her chances, Robin wanted to know. Should they put her through yet more of this? Or should they take her home and let her die?

Many talk about the border between what we can do and what we can't as if it were a bright line drawn across the hospital bed. Analysts often note how ridiculous it is that we spend more than a quarter of public health care dollars on the last six months of life. Perhaps we could spare this fruitless spending—if only we knew when people's last six months would be.

In the absence of certainty, the truth is we want doctors who fight. Through a friend, I met Watson Bowes Jr., a nationally known professor of obstetrics, now emeritus, from the University of North Carolina. We got talking and I asked him what he was most proud of in his career. I expected to hear about laboratory discoveries or obstetric techniques. He had done foundational research on how oxygen is carried to the fetus, and he had been among the first in America to learn how to give blood transfusions to fetuses. But what made him most proud, he told me, was an experiment he had done as a young obstetrician at the University of Colorado in 1975. At that time, babies born two months prematurely or more were considered to have almost no chance to survive. Little, therefore, was done for them. For one year, however, he decided to treat those babies as if they would live—no matter how blue, how weak, how small. The doctors on his team used no new technologies. They simply did everything they would normally do for a full-term baby. If the baby had trouble in delivery, they did a C-section, when before they would have spared a mother the surgery for such a hopeless child. They used fetal heart monitors when they usually wouldn't have. They put in intravenous lines and placed the babies on respirators, however limp and lifeless they seemed. And they discovered that the vast majority of these premature babies, babies only two or three pounds in size, could survive to be normal and healthy—just by the doctors' fighting for them.

Even when we don't know that a patient can be completely normal and healthy, we want doctors to fight. Consider again the wars in Iraq and Afghanistan, where military surgeons have learned how to save soldiers who have never been saved before—soldiers with almost a hundred percent of their bodies burned, soldiers with severe and permanent head injuries, soldiers who have had abdominal injuries and three limbs blown away. We have no idea whether it is possible to live a good life with no arms and only one leg. But we don't want the doctors to give up. Instead, we want them to consider it their task to learn how to rehabilitate survivors despite the unprecedented severity of their injuries. We want doctors to push and find a way.

We also want doctors to fight even in the most mundane of situations. My ten-year-old daughter, Hattie, has had to deal with severe psoriasis for a long time. It is hardly life-threatening. But the condition has left her with thick red itchy and scaling patches all over—on her knees, her back, her scalp, her face. The dermatologist tried stronger and stronger steroid creams and medications. These damped the disease down somewhat, but only some of the angry patches went away. This was about as good as we could do for her, he said. We would just try to control the disease and hope Hattie outgrew it. So for a long while we lived with her condition. But she hated it, and she hated the eruptions on her face most of all. She kept asking her mother and me, "Please, just take me to another doctor." So finally we did. The second dermatologist said she had something else she wanted to try. She put Hattie on amoxicillin, an ordinary antibiotic. It doesn't work in adults, she said, but sometimes it does in kids. In two weeks, the patches were gone.

The seemingly easiest and most sensible rule for a doctor to follow is: Always Fight. Always look for what more you could do. I am sympathetic to this rule. It gives us our best chance of avoiding the worst error of all—giving up on someone we could have helped.

I have a friend whose elderly grandmother went into shock from gastric bleeding from taking ibuprofen for a backache. The bleeding was torrential. She had to be given multiple blood transfusions just to keep up with the hemorrhaging. The units of packed red cells and plasma were put in pressure bags to pump them into her frail veins as quickly as possible. She underwent emergency endoscopies and angiograms, and after many hours of effort the bleeding vessel was found and stopped. But she did not do well afterwards. She remained in intensive care for weeks, unconscious, on a ventilator. Her lungs and heart went into failure. She eventually required a tracheostomy, a feeding tube, an arterial line in one arm, central venous lines in her neck, and a urinary catheter. More than a month went by with no sign of improvement. The family agonized about keeping on with the treatment. The likelihood of her recovering a life she would find worth living seemed dismal. Eventually, the family went to the doctors and told them they had decided it was time to withdraw life support.

But the doctors balked. Let's wait a while longer, they said. "They were solicitous but quite firm," my friend says. They didn't want to hear about stopping. So the family bowed to their will. And ten days or so later, my friend's grandmother began to improve dramatically. The team was soon able to remove her tubes. Her tracheotomy healed over. She turned the corner, and although it took still more weeks of recovery, she got back to her life and enjoyed it for several years after. "She told me repeatedly how glad she was to be here," he says.

So maybe we should never hold back, never stop pushing. In the face of uncertainty, what could be safer? It doesn't take long to realize, however, that the rule is neither viable nor humane. All doctors—whether surgeons, psychiatrists, or dermatologists—have patients they are unable to heal, or even to diagnose, no matter how hard they try. I have several patients who have come to me with chronic, severe abdominal pain of one sort or another. And I have tried all I can to figure out the cause of their pain. I have done CT scans and MRIs. I have sent the patients to gastroenterologists, who endoscoped their colons and their stomachs. I have ruled out pancreatitis, gastritis, ulcers, lactose intolerance, and lesser known conditions like celiac sprue. But their pain has remained. Just take out my gallbladder, one patient pleaded with me, and even her internist joined in. The pain was in the exact location of her gallbladder. But the gallbladder looked normal on all the tests. So do you take out the gallbladder on the off chance it is the source? At some point you have to admit that you are up against a problem you are not going to solve and that, by pushing further and harder, you might well do more harm than good. Sometimes there is nothing you can do.

I was walking down the hallway one day, when Jeanne, one of the intensive care unit nurses, stopped me, visibly angry. "What is it with you doctors?" she said. "Don't you ever know when to stop?" That day she'd been caring for a man with lung cancer. He had had one of his lungs removed and had been in intensive care for all but three weeks of the five months since. A pneumonia that blossomed in his remaining lung early after surgery had left him unable to breathe without a tracheostomy and a respirator. He had to be heavily sedated or else his oxygen levels dropped. He received nutrition through a surgically placed gastric tube. Sepsis claimed his kidneys and the team put him on continuous dialysis. It had long ago become apparent that a life outside the hospital was not possible for this man. But neither the doctors nor his wife seemed capable of confronting this truth—because he did not have a terminal disease (his cancer had been removed successfully) and he was only in his fifties. So there he lay, with no evident hope of progress and his doctors simply trying to keep him from falling back. This was not the only patient Jeanne had like this, either.

But as we talked, Jeanne also told me of doctors she thought had stopped pushing too soon. So I asked what she felt the best doctors did. She thought for a while before answering. Good doctors, she finally said, understand one key thing: "This is not about them. It's about the patient." The good doctors didn't always get the answers right, she said.

Sometimes they still pushed too long or not long enough. But at least they stopped to wonder, to reconsider the path they were on. They asked colleagues for another perspective. They set aside their egos.

This insight is wiser and harder to grasp than it might seem. When someone has come to you for your expertise and your expertise has failed, what do you have left? You have only your character to fall back upon—and sometimes it's only your pride that comes through. You may simply deny your plan has failed, deny that more can't be done. You may become angry. You may blame the person—"She didn't follow my instructions!" You may dread just seeing that person again. I have done all these things. But they never come to any good.

In the end, no guidelines can tell us what we have power over and what we don't. In the face of uncertainty, wisdom is to err on the side of pushing, to not give up. But you have to be ready to recognize when pushing is only ego, only weakness. You have to be ready to recognize when the pushing can turn to harm.

In a way, our task *is* to "Always Fight." But our fight is not always to do more. It is to do right by our patients, even though what is right is not always clear.

CALLIE'S DOCTORS COULD not say exactly how slim her chances were once the rounds of chemotherapy had failed. Who knew what an experimental drug or a yet different chemotherapy could do? There were still possibilities for success. But her doctors also made sure that Callie and her parents knew that it was all right if they wanted to stop.

As I talked to Robin, her father, who was in agony and trying to understand what should be done, I found I could do little more than confirm the choices her doctors had laid out. He wanted hope that his daughter would live. But he did not want to subject her to fruitless suffering. If a further treatment could save two in a hundred children but would subject ninety-eight of them to a painful death, would that treatment be worth trying for Callie? I had no answer. Callie and her parents were left to sort through the questions by themselves.

Not long after we spoke, Callie's mother, Shelley, sent an e-mail to relatives and friends that began with a quotation. " 'We must eradicate from the soul all fear and terror of what comes to us out of the future,' " it said. Two days later, on April 7, 2006, Callie's parents brought her home. On April 17, Shelley wrote again: "Callie died peacefully at home shortly after 1 A.M. Easter Monday. We are all fine. Our home is filled with incredible peace."

Part III

Ingenuity

The Score

At 5:00 A.M. on a cool Boston morning not long ago, Elizabeth Rourke—thick black-brown hair, pale Irish skin, and forty-one weeks pregnant—reached over and woke her husband, Chris.

"I'm having contractions," she said.

"Are you sure?" he asked.

"I'm sure."

She was a week past her due date, and the pain was deep and viselike, nothing like the occasional spasms she'd been feeling. It seemed to come out of her lower back and to wrap around and seize her whole abdomen. The first spasm woke her out of sound sleep. Then a second came. And a third.

She was carrying their first child. So far, the pregnancy

had gone well, aside from the exhaustion and the nausea of the first trimester, when all she felt like doing was lying on the couch watching *Law & Order* reruns. ("I can't look at Sam Waterston anymore without feeling kind of ill," she says.) An internist who had just finished her residency, she had landed a job at the Massachusetts General Hospital a few months before and managed to work until she was full term. She and her husband now sat up in bed, timing the spasms by the clock on the bedside table. They were seven minutes apart, and they stayed that way for a while.

Rourke called her obstetrician's office at 8:30, when the phones were turned on, but she knew what the people there were going to say: Don't come to the hospital until the contractions are five minutes apart and last at least a minute. "You take the childbirth class, and they drill it into you a million times," Rourke says. "The whole point of childbirth classes, as far as I could tell, was to make sure you keep your butt out of the hospital until you're really in labor."

The nurse asked if the contractions were five minutes apart and lasted more than a minute. No. Had she broken her water? No. Well, she had a "good start." But she should wait to come in.

During her medical training, Rourke had seen about fifty births and delivered four babies herself. The last birth she had seen was in a hospital parking lot.

"They had called, saying, 'We're delivering! We're coming to the hospital, and she's delivering!'" Rourke says. "So we were in the ER and we went running. It was freezing cold. The car came screeching up to the hospital. The door went flying open. And, sure enough, there the mom was. We could see the baby's head. The resident running next to me got there a second before I did, and he puts his arms down, and the baby went—*phhhoom*—straight into his arms in the middle of the parking lot. It was freezing cold outside, and I'll never forget the steam pouring off the baby. It's blue and crying and the steam was pouring off of it. Then we put this tiny little baby on this enormous stretcher and raced it back into the hospital."

Rourke didn't want to deliver in a parking lot. She wanted a nice, normal vaginal delivery. She didn't even want an epidural. "I didn't want to be confined to bed," she says. "I didn't want to be dead from the waist down. I didn't want a urinary catheter to have to be put in. Everything about the epidural was totally unappealing to me." She was not afraid of the pain. Having seen how too many deliveries had gone, she was mainly afraid of losing her ability to control what was done to her.

She had considered hiring a doula—a birthing coach—to stay with her through delivery. There are studies showing that having a doula can lower the likelihood a mother will end up with a Cesarean section or an epidural. The more she looked into it, however, the more worried she became about being paired with someone annoying. She thought about delivering with a midwife. But, as a doctor, she felt that she would have more control working with another doctor.

She was not feeling very much in control at the moment, though. By midday, her contractions hadn't really speeded up; they were still coming every seven minutes, maybe every six minutes at most. She was finding it increasingly difficult to get comfortable. "The way it felt best was, strangely enough, to be on all fours," she recalls. So she just hung around the house like that—on all fours during the contractions, her husband close by, both of them nervous and giddy about their baby being on the way.

Finally, at 4:30 in the afternoon, the contractions began coming five minutes apart, and they set off in their Jetta, with the infant car seat installed in the back, her bag packed with everything that *The Girlfriends' Guide to Pregnancy* said to bring, right down to the lipstick (which she doesn't even wear). When they reached the hospital admissions desk, she was ready. Their baby was on the way, and she was eager to bring it into the world as nature had intended.

"I wanted no intervention, no doctors, no drugs. I didn't want any of that stuff," she says. "In a perfect world, I wanted to have my baby in a forest bower attended by fairy sprites."

HUMAN BIRTH IS an astonishing natural phenomenon. Carol Burnett once told Bill Cosby how he could understand what the experience was like. "Take your bottom lip and pull it as far away from your face as you can," she said. "Now pull it over your head." The process is a solution to an evolutionary problem: how a mammal can walk upright, which requires a small, fixed, bony pelvis, and also possess a large brain, which entails a baby whose head is too big to fit through that small pelvis. Part of the solution is that, in a sense, all human mothers give birth prematurely. Other mammals are born mature enough to walk and seek food within hours; our newborns are small and helpless for months. Even so, human birth is a feat involving an intricate sequence of events.

First, a mother's pelvis enlarges. Starting in the first trimester, maternal hormones stretch and loosen the joints holding the four bones of the pelvis together. Almost an inch of space is added. Pregnant women sometimes feel the different parts of their pelvis moving when they walk.

Then, when it's time for delivery, the uterus changes. During gestation, it's a snug, rounded, hermetically sealed pouch; during labor it takes on the shape of a funnel. And each contraction pushes the baby's head down through that funnel, into the pelvis. This happens even in paraplegic women; the mother does not have to do anything.

Meanwhile, the cervix—which is, through pregnancy, a rigid, more-than-inch-thick cylinder of muscle and connective tissue capping the end of the funnel—softens and relaxes. Pressure from the baby's head gradually stretches the tissue until it is paper-thin—a process known as "effacement." A small circular opening appears, and each contraction widens it, like a tight shirt being pulled over a child's head. Until the contractions pull the cervix open about four inches, or ten centimeters—the full temple-to-temple diameter of the child's head—the child cannot get out. So the state of the cervix determines when birth will occur. At two or three centimeters of dilation, a mother is still in "early" labor. Delivery is many hours away. At four to seven centimeters, the contractions grow stronger. "Active" labor has begun. At some point, the amniotic sac surrounding the fetus breaks under the pressure, and the clear fluid gushes out. Contractile force increases further.

At between seven and ten centimeters of cervical dilation, the "transition phase," the contractions reach their greatest intensity. The contractions press the baby's head into the vagina and the narrowest part of the pelvis's bony ring. The pelvis is usually wider from side to side than front to back, so it's best if the baby emerges with the temples—the widest portion of the head—lined up side to side with the mother's pelvis. The top of the head comes into view. The mother has a mounting urge to push. The head comes out, then the shoulders, and suddenly a breathing, wailing child is born. The umbilical cord is cut. The placenta separates from the uterine lining, and with a slight tug on the cord and a push from the mother, it is extruded. The uterus spontaneously contracts into a clenched ball of muscle, closing off its bleeding sinuses—the expanded veins in the uterine wall. Typically, the mother's breasts immediately let down with colostrum, the first milk, and the newborn can latch on to feed.

That's if all goes well. At almost any step, the process can go wrong. For thousands of years, childbirth was the most common cause of death for young women and infants. There's the risk of hemorrhage. The placenta can tear or separate, or a portion may remain stuck in the uterus after delivery and then bleed torrentially. Or the uterus may not contract after delivery, so that the raw surfaces and sinuses keep bleeding until the mother dies of blood loss. Sometimes the uterus ruptures during labor.

Infection can set in. Once the water breaks, the chances that bacteria will get into the uterus rise with each passing hour. During the nineteenth century, as Semmelweis discovered, doctors often introduced infection, because they examined more infected patients than midwives did and because they failed to wash their contaminated hands. Bacteria routinely invaded and killed the fetus and, often, the mother with it. Puerperal fever remained the leading cause of maternal death in the era before antibiotics. Even today, if a mother doesn't deliver within twenty-four hours after her water breaks, she has a 40 percent chance of becoming infected.

The most basic problem is "obstruction of labor"—not being able to get the baby out. The baby may be too big, especially when pregnancy continues beyond the fortieth week. The mother's pelvis may be too small, as was frequently the case when lack of vitamin D and calcium made rickets common. The baby might arrive at the birth canal sideways, with nothing but an arm sticking out. It could be a breech, coming butt first and getting stuck with its legs up on its chest. It could be a footling breech, coming feet first but then getting wedged at the chest with the arms above the head. It could come out headfirst but get stuck because its head is turned the wrong way. Sometimes the head makes it out, but the shoulders get stuck behind the pubic bone of the mother's pelvis.

These situations are dangerous. When a baby is stuck, the umbilical cord, the only source of fetal blood and oxygen, eventually becomes trapped or compressed, causing the baby to asphyxiate. Mothers have sometimes labored for astonishing lengths of time, unable to deliver, and died with their child in the process. In 1817, for example, Princess Charlotte of Wales, King George IV's twenty-one-year-old daughter, spent four days in labor. Her nine-pound boy was in a sideways position with a head too large for Charlotte's pelvis. Only after the fiftieth hour of active labor did he finally emerge—stillborn. Six hours later, Charlotte herself died, from hemorrhagic shock. As she was George's only child, the throne passed to his brother instead of her, then to his niece—which is how Victoria became queen.

Midwives and doctors long sought ways out of such disasters, and the history of ingenuity in obstetrics is the history of these efforts. The first reliably lifesaving invention for mothers was called a crochet, or, in another variation, a cranioclast: a long, sharply pointed instrument, often with clawlike hooks, which birth attendants used in desperate situations to perforate and crush a fetus's skull, extract the fetus, and save, at least, the mother's life.

Many obstetricians and midwives made their names by devising ways to get both a mother and baby through obstructed deliveries. There is, for example, the Lovset maneuver for a breech baby with its arms trapped above the head: you take the baby by the hips and turn it sideways, then reach in, take an upper arm, and sweep it down over the chest and out. If a breech baby's arms are out but the head is trapped, you have the Mariceau-Smellie-Veit maneuver: you place your finger in the baby's mouth, which allows you to pull forcefully while still controlling the head.

The child with its head out but a shoulder stuck—a "shoulder dystocia"—will asphyxiate within five to seven minutes unless it is freed and delivered. Sometimes sharp downward pressure with a fist just above the mother's pubic bone can dislodge the shoulder; if not, there is the Woods corkscrew maneuver, in which you reach in, grab the baby's posterior shoulder, and push it backward to free the child. There's also the Rubin maneuver (you grab the stuck, anterior shoulder and push it forward toward the baby's chest to release it) and the McRoberts maneuver (sharply flex the mother's legs up onto her abdomen and so lift her pubic bone off the baby's shoulder). Finally, there is the maneuver that no one wanted to put his name to but that has saved many babies' lives through history: you fracture the clavicles—the collar bones—and pull the baby out.

There are dozens of these maneuvers, and, though they have saved the lives of countless babies, each has a significant failure rate. Surgery has been known since ancient times as a way to save an entrapped baby. Roman law in the seventh century B.C. forbade burial of an undelivered woman until the child had been cut out, in the hope that the child would survive. In 1614, Pope Paul V issued a similar edict, ordering that the child be baptized if it was still alive. But Cesarean section on a living mother was considered criminal for much of history, because it almost always killed the mother—through hemorrhage and infection—and her life took precedence over that of the child. (The name "Cesarean" section may have arisen from the tale that Caesar was born of his mother, Aurelia, by an abdominal delivery, but historians regard the story as a myth, since Aurelia lived long after his birth.) Only after the development, in the late nineteenth century, of anesthesia and antisepsis and, in the early twentieth century, of a double-layer suturing technique that could stop an opened uterus from hemorrhaging, did Cesarean section become a real option. Even then, it was held in low repute. And that was because a better option was around: the obstetrical forceps.

The story of the forceps is both extraordinary and disturbing, because it is the story of a lifesaving idea that was kept secret for more than century. The instrument was developed by Peter Chamberlen (1575–1628), the first of a long line of French Huguenots who delivered babies in London. It looked like a pair of big metal salad tongs, with two blades shaped to fit snugly around a baby's head and handles that locked together with a single screw in the middle. It let doctors more or less yank stuck babies out and, carefully applied, was the first technique that could save both the baby and the mother. The Chamberlens knew they were onto something, and they resolved to keep the device a family secret. Whenever they were called in to help with a mother in obstructed labor, they ushered everyone else out of the room and covered the mother's lower half with a sheet or a blanket so that even she couldn't see what was going on. They kept the secret of the forceps for three generations. In 1670, Hugh Chamberlen, in the third generation, tried and failed to sell the design to the French government. Late in his life, he divulged it to an Amsterdam-based obstetrician, Roger Roonhuysen, who kept the technique within his own family for sixty more years. The secret did not get out until the mid-eighteenth century. Once it did, it gained wide acceptance. At the time of Princess Charlotte's failed delivery in 1817, her obstetrician, Sir Richard Croft, was widely reviled for failing to use forceps to assist. In remorse for her death, he shot himself to death not long afterward.

By the early twentieth century, the problems of human birth seemed to have been largely solved. Doctors could avail themselves of a range of measures to ensure a safe delivery: antiseptics, the forceps, blood transfusions, a drug (ergot) that could induce labor and contract the uterus after delivery to stop bleeding, and even, in desperate situations, Cesarean section. By the 1930s, most urban mothers had shifted from mid-wife deliveries at home to physician deliveries in the hospital.

But in 1933 the New York Academy of Medicine pub-lished a shocking study of 2,041 maternal deaths in childbirth in New York City. At least two-thirds, the investigators found, were preventable. There had been no improvement in death rates for mothers in the preceding two decades; death rates for newborns had actually increased. Hospital care brought no ad-vantages; mothers were better off delivering at home. The in-vestigators were appalled to find that many physicians simply didn't know what they were doing: they missed clear signs of hemorrhagic shock and other treatable conditions, violated basic antiseptic standards, tore and infected women with mis-applied forceps. The White House followed with a similar na-tional report. Doctors may have had the right tools, but midwives without them did better.

The two reports brought modern obstetrics to a critical turning point. Specialists in the field had shown extraordinary ingenuity. They had developed the knowledge and instrumen-tation to solve many problems of child delivery. Yet knowl-edge and instrumentation had proved grossly insufficient. If obstetrics wasn't to go the way of phrenology or trepanning, it had to discover a different kind of ingenuity. It had to figure out how to standardize childbirth.

Three-quarters of a century later, the degree to which birth has been transformed by medicine is astounding and, for some, alarming. Today, electronic fetal heart-rate monitoring is used in more than 90 percent of deliveries, intravenous flu-ids in more than 80 percent, epidural anesthesia in three-quarters, medicines to speed up labor (the drug of choice is no longer ergot but Pitocin, a synthetic form of the natural hormone that drives contractions) in at least half. Thirty percent of American deliveries are now by Cesarean section, and that proportion continues to rise. The field of obstetrics has changed—and, perhaps irreversibly, so has childbirth itself.

AN ADMITTING CLERK led Elizabeth Rourke and her husband into a small triage room. A nurse midwife timed her contractions—they were indeed five minutes apart—and then did a pelvic examination to see how dilated Rourke was. After twelve hours of regular, painful contractions, Rourke figured that she might be at seven or eight centimeters. Instead, she was at two.

It was disheartening news: her labor was only just starting. The nurse practitioner thought about sending her home but eventually decided to admit her. The labor floor was a horseshoe of twelve patient rooms strung around a nurses' station. For hospitals, deliveries are a good business. If mothers have a positive experience, they stay loyal to the hospital for years. So the rooms are made to seem as warm and inviting as possible for what is, essentially, a procedure room. Each has recessed lighting, decorator window curtains, comfortable chairs for the family, individualized climate control. Rourke's even had a Jacuzzi. She spent the next several hours soaking in the tub, sitting on a rubber birthing ball, or walking the halls—stopping to brace herself with each contraction.

By 10:30 that night, the contractions had sped up, coming every two minutes. The doctor on duty for her obstetrician's group performed a pelvic examination. Her cervix was still only two centimeters dilated: the labor had stalled, if it had ever really started.

The doctor gave her two options. She could have active labor induced with Pitocin. Or she could go home, rest, and wait for true active labor to begin. Rourke did not like the idea of using the drug. So at midnight she and her husband went home.

No sooner was she home than she realized that she had made a mistake. The pain was too much. Chris had conked out on the bed, and she couldn't get through this on her own. She held out for another two and a half hours, just to avoid looking foolish, and then got Chris to drive her back. At 2:43 A.M., the nurse scanned her in again—she was still wearing her bar-coded hospital identification bracelet. The obstetrician re-examined her. Rourke was nearly four centimeters dilated. She had progressed to active labor.

Rourke began to feel her will fading, however. She had been having regular contractions for twenty-two hours and was exhausted from sleeplessness and pain. She tried a narcotic called Nubain to dull the pain, and when that didn't work, she broke down and asked for an epidural. An anesthesiologist came in and had her sit on the side of the bed with her back to him. She felt a cold, wet swipe of antiseptic along her spine, the pressure of a needle, and a twinge that shot down her leg; the epidural catheter was in. The doctor gave a bolus of local anesthetic into the tubing, and the pain of the contractions melted away into numbness. Then her blood pressure dropped—a known side effect of epidural injections. The team poured fluids into her intravenously and gave injections of ephedrine to increase her—and her baby's—blood pressure.

It took fifteen minutes to stabilize her blood pressure. But the monitor showed that the baby's heart rate remained normal the whole time, about 150 beats a minute. The team dispersed and around 4:00 A.M., Rourke fell asleep.

At 6:00 A.M., the obstetrician returned and, to Rourke's dismay, found her still just four centimeters dilated. Her determination to avoid medical interventions ebbed further, and a Pitocin drip was started. The contractions surged. At 7:30 A.M., she was six centimeters dilated. This was real progress. Rourke was elated. She rested some more. She felt her strength coming back. She readied herself to start pushing in a few hours.

Dr. Alessandra Peccei took over with the new day and looked at the whiteboard behind the nursing station where the hourly progress of the mother in each room is recorded. In a typical morning, a mother in one room might have been pushing while a mother in another was having her labor induced with medication; in still another, a mother might be just waiting, her cervix only partially dilated and the baby still high. Rourke was a "G2P0 41.2 wks pit+ 6/100/-2" on the whiteboard—a mother with two gestations, zero born (Rourke had had a previous miscarriage), forty-one weeks and two days pregnant. She was on Pitocin. Her cervix was six centimeters dilated and 100 percent effaced. The baby was at negative-two station, which is about seven centimeters from crowning, that is, from becoming visible at the vaginal orifice.

Peccei went into Rourke's room and introduced herself as the attending obstetrician. Peccei, who was forty-two years old and had delivered more than two thousand newborns, projected a comforting combination of competence and friendliness. She had given birth to her own children with a midwife. Rourke felt that they understood each other.

Peccei waited three hours to allow Rourke's labor to progress. At 10:30 A.M., she reexamined her and frowned. The cervix was unchanged, still six centimeters dilated. The baby had not come down any further. Peccei felt along the top of the baby's head for the soft spot in back to get a sense of which way it was facing and found it facing sideways. The baby was stuck.

Sometimes increasing the strength of the contractions can turn the baby's head in the right direction and push it along. So, using a gloved finger, Peccei punctured the bulging membrane of Rourke's amniotic sac. The waters burst out, and immediately the contractions picked up strength and speed. The baby did not budge, however. Worse, on the monitor, its heart rate began to drop with each contraction—120, 100, 80, it went, taking almost a minute before recovering to normal. It's not always clear what dips like these mean. Malpractice lawyers like to say that they are a baby's "cry for help." In some cases, they are. An abnormal tracing can signal that a baby is getting an inadequate supply of oxygen or blood—the baby's cord might be wrapped around its neck or getting squeezed off altogether. But usually, even when the baby's heart rate takes a prolonged dive, lasting well past the end of a contraction, the baby is fine. A drop in heart rate is often simply what happens when a baby's head is squeezed really hard.

Dr. Peccei couldn't be sure which was the case. So she turned off the Pitocin drip, to reduce the strength of the contractions. She gave Rourke, and therefore the baby, extra oxygen by nasal prong. She scratched at the baby's scalp to irritate it and make sure the baby's heart rate responded. The heart rate continued to drop during contractions, but it never failed to recover. After twenty-five minutes, the decelerations finally disappeared. The baby's heart rate was back to being steadily normal.

Now what? Rourke had not dilated any further in five hours. The baby's head was stuck sideways. She'd been in labor for thirty hours to this point, and her baby didn't seem to be going anywhere.

THERE ARE 130,000,000 births around the world each year, more than 4,000,000 of them in the United States. No matter what is done, some percentage are going to end badly. All the same, physicians have had an abiding faith that they could step in and at least reduce that percentage. When the national reports of the 1930s proved that obstetrics had failed to do so and that incompetence was an important reason, the medical profession turned to a strategy of instituting strict regulations on individual practice. Training requirements were established for physicians delivering babies. Hospitals set firm rules about who could do deliveries, what steps they had to follow, and whether they would be permitted to use forceps and other risky interventions. Hospital and state authorities investigated maternal deaths for aberrations from basic standards.

Having these standards reduced maternal deaths substantially. In the mid-1930s, delivering a child had been the single most dangerous event in a woman's life: one in 150 pregnancies ended in the death of the mother. By the 1950s, owing in part to the tighter standards and in part to the discovery of penicillin and other antibiotics, the risk of death for a mother had fallen more than 90 percent, to just one in two thousand.

But the situation wasn't so encouraging for newborns: one in thirty still died at birth—odds that were scarcely better than they were a century before—and it wasn't clear how that could be changed. Then a doctor named Virginia Apgar, who was working in New York, had an idea. It was a ridiculously simple idea, but it transformed childbirth and the care of the newly born. Apgar was an unlikely revolutionary for obstetrics. For starters, she had never delivered a baby—not as a doctor and not even as a mother.

Apgar was one of the first women to be admitted to the surgical residency at Columbia University College of Physicians and Surgeons, in 1933. The daughter of a Westfield, New Jersey, insurance executive, she was tall and would have been imposing if not for her horn-rimmed glasses and bobby pins. She had a combination of fearlessness, warmth, and natural enthusiasm that drew people to her. When anyone was having troubles, she would sit down and say, "Tell Momma all about it." At the same time, she was exacting about everything she did. She wasn't just a talented violinist; she also made her own instruments. She began flying single-engine planes at the age of fifty-nine. When she was a resident, a patient she had operated on died after surgery. "Virginia worried and worried that she might have clamped a small but essential artery," Stanley James, a colleague of hers, later recalled. "No autopsy permit could be obtained. So she secretly went to the morgue and opened the operative incision to find the cause. That small artery had been clamped. She immediately told the surgeon. She never tried to cover a mistake. She had to know the truth no matter what the cost."

At the end of her surgical residency, her chairman told her that, however good she was, a female surgeon had little chance of attracting patients. He persuaded her to join Columbia's faculty as an anesthesiologist, which was then a position of far lesser status. She threw herself into the job, becoming the second woman in the country to be board certified in anesthesiology. She established anesthesia as its own division at Columbia and, eventually, as its own department, on an equal footing with surgery. She administered anesthesia to more than twenty thousand patients during her career. She even carried a scalpel and a length of tubing in her purse, in case a passerby needed an emergency airway—and apparently employed them successfully more than a dozen times. "Do what is right and do it now," she used to say.

Throughout her career, the work she loved most was providing anesthesia for child deliveries. She loved the renewal of a new child's coming into the world. But she was appalled by the care that many newborns received. Babies who were born malformed or too small or just blue and not breathing well were listed as stillborn, placed out of sight, and left to die. They were believed to be too sick to live. Apgar believed otherwise, but she had no authority to challenge the conventions. She was not an obstetrician, and she was a female in a male world. So she took a less direct but ultimately more powerful approach: she devised a score.

The Apgar score, as it became universally known, allowed nurses to rate the condition of babies at birth on a scale from zero to ten. An infant got two points if it was pink all over, two for crying, two for taking good, vigorous breaths, two for moving all four limbs, and two if its heart rate was over a hundred. Ten points meant a child born in perfect condition. Four points or less meant a blue, limp baby.

Published in 1953 to revolutionary effect, the score turned an intangible and impressionistic clinical concept—the condition of new babies—into numbers that people could collect and compare. Using it required more careful observation and documentation of the true condition of every baby. Moreover, even if only because doctors are competitive, it drove them to want to produce better scores—and therefore better outcomes—for the newborns they delivered.

Around the world, virtually every child born in a hospital came to have an Apgar score recorded at one minute after birth and at five minutes after birth. It quickly became clear that a baby with a terrible Apgar score at one minute could often be resuscitated—with measures like oxygen and warming—to an excellent score at five minutes. Neonatal intensive care units sprang into existence. The score also began to alter how childbirth itself was managed. Spinal and then epidural anesthesia were found to produce babies with better scores than general anesthesia. Prenatal ultrasound came into use to detect problems for deliveries in advance. Fetal heart monitors became standard. Over the years, hundreds of adjustments and innovations in care were made, resulting in what's sometimes called "the obstetrics package." And that package has produced dramatic results. In the United States today, a full-term baby dies in just one childbirth out of five hundred, and a mother dies in less than one in ten thousand. If the statistics of

1930 had persisted, 27,000 mothers would have died last year (instead of fewer than five hundred)—and 160,000 newborns (instead of one-eighth that number).

THERE'S A PARADOX here. Ask most research physicians how a profession can advance, and they will tell you about the model of "evidence-based medicine"—the idea that nothing ought to be introduced into practice unless it has been properly tested and proved effective by research centers, preferably through a double blind, randomized controlled trial. But in a 1978 ranking of medical specialties according to their use of hard evidence from randomized clinical trials, obstetrics came in last. Obstetricians did few randomized trials, and when they did they largely ignored the results. Take fetal heart monitors. Careful studies have found that they provide no added benefit in routine labors over having nurses simply listen to the baby's heart rate hourly. In fact, the use of monitors seems to increase unnecessary Cesarean sections, because slight abnormalities in the tracings make everyone nervous about waiting for vaginal delivery. Nonetheless, they are used in nearly all hospital child deliveries. Or consider the virtual disappearance of forceps in the delivery wards, even though several studies have compared forceps delivery to Cesarean section and found no advantage for Cesarean section. (A few found that mothers actually did better with forceps.)

Doctors in other fields have always looked down their masked noses on their obstetrical colleagues. They didn't think they were very smart—obstetricians long had trouble attracting the top medical students to their specialty—and there seemed little science or sophistication to what they did. Yet almost nothing else in medicine has saved lives on the scale that obstetrics has. Yes, there have been dazzling changes in what we can do to treat disease and improve people's lives. We now have drugs to stop strokes and to treat cancers; we have coronary artery stents, mechanical joints, and artificial respirators. But do those of us in other fields of medicine use these measures anywhere near as reliably and as safely as obstetricians use theirs? We don't come close.

Ordinary pneumonia, for instance, remains the fourth most common cause of death in affluent countries, and the death rate has actually worsened in the past quarter century. That's in part because pneumonias have become more severe, but it's also because we doctors haven't performed all that well. Elegant research trials have shown us the best antibiotics to use and that patients needing hospitalization are less likely to die if the antibiotics are started within four hours of arrival. But we pay little attention to what actually happens in practice. A recent study has concluded that 40 percent of pneumonia patients do not get the antibiotics on time. When we do give the antibiotics, 20 percent of patients get the wrong kind.

In obstetrics, meanwhile, if a new strategy seemed worth trying, doctors did not wait for research trials to tell them if it was all right. They just went ahead and tried it, then looked to see if results improved. Obstetrics went about improving the same way Toyota and General Electric went about improving: on the fly, but always paying attention to the results and trying to better them. And that approach worked. Whether all the adjustments and innovations of the obstetrics package are necessary and beneficial may remain unclear—routine fetal heart monitoring is still controversial, for example. But the package as a whole has made child delivery demonstrably safer, and it has done so despite the increasing age, obesity, and consequent health problems of pregnant mothers.

The Apgar score changed everything. It was practical and easy to calculate, and it gave clinicians at the bedside immediate feedback on how effective their care was. In the rest of medicine, we are used to measuring dozens of specific things: blood counts, electrolyte levels, heart rates, viral titers. But we have no routine measure that puts the data together to grade how the patient as a whole is faring. We have only an impression of how we're performing—and sometimes not even that. At the end of a difficult operation, have I given my patient a one in fifty chance of death, or one in five hundred? I cannot say. I have no feel for the difference along the way. "How did the surgery go?" the patient's family will ask me. "Fine," I can only say.

The Apgar effect wasn't just a matter of giving clinicians a quick objective read of how they had done. The score also changed the choices they made about how to do better. Chiefs of obstetrics services began poring over the Apgar results of their doctors and midwives, and by doing so they became no different from the bread factory floor manager taking stock of how many loaves the bakers burned. They both want solutions that will lift the results of every employee, from the most novice to the most experienced. That means sometimes choosing reliability over the possibility of occasional perfection.

The fate of the forceps is a revealing example. I spoke to Watson Bowes Jr., the University of North Carolina emeritus professor of obstetrics, about what happened to the forceps.

In addition to his studies on the care of premature babies, he was the author of a widely read textbook chapter on forceps technique. He had also practiced in the 1960s, when less than 5 percent of deliveries were by C-section and more than 40 percent were with forceps. Yes, he said, many studies showed fabulous results for forceps. But they only showed how well forceps deliveries could go in the hands of very experienced obstetricians at large hospitals. Meanwhile, the profession was being held responsible for improving Apgar scores and mortality rates for newborns everywhere—at hospitals small and large, with doctors of all levels of experience.

"Forceps deliveries are very difficult to teach—much more difficult than a C-section," Bowes said. "With a C-section, you stand across from the learner. You can see exactly what they're doing. You can say, 'Not there. *There.*' With the forceps, though, there is a feel that is very hard to teach."

Just putting the forceps on a baby's head is tricky. You have to choose the right type for the shape of the mother's pelvis and the size of the child's head—and there are at least half a dozen types of forceps. You have to slide the blades symmetrically along the sides, traveling exactly in the space between the ears and the eyes and over the cheekbones. "For most residents, it took two or three years of training to get this consistently right," he said. Then a doctor must apply forces of both traction and compression—pulling, Bowes's chapter explained, with an average of forty to seventy pounds of axial force and five pounds of fetal skull compression. "When you put tension on the forceps, you should have some sense that there is movement," he said. Too much force and skin can tear, the skull can fracture, a fatal brain hemorrhage may result. "Some residents had a real feel for it," Bowes said. "Others didn't."

The question facing obstetrics was this: Is medicine a craft or an industry? If medicine is a craft, then you focus on teaching obstetricians to acquire a set of artisanal skills—the Woods corkscrew maneuver for the baby with a shoulder stuck, the Lovset maneuver for the breech baby, the feel of a forceps for a baby whose head is too big. You do research to find new techniques. You accept that things will not always work out in everyone's hands.

But if medicine is an industry, responsible for the safest possible delivery of some four million babies a year in the United States alone, then a new understanding is required. The focus shifts. You seek reliability. You begin to wonder whether forty-two thousand obstetricians in the Unites States could really safely master all these techniques. You notice the steady reports of terrible forceps injuries to babies and mothers, despite all the training that clinicians received. After Apgar, obstetricians decided that they needed a simpler, more predictable way to intervene when a laboring mother ran into trouble. They found it in the Cesarean section.

JUST AFTER 7:30 P.M., in the thirty-ninth hour of her labor, Elizabeth Rourke underwent surgery to deliver her baby. Peccei had offered her the option of a Cesarean eight hours before, but Rourke refused. She hadn't been ready to give up on pushing her little baby out into the world, and, though the doctor doubted Rourke's efforts would succeed, the baby was doing fine on the heart monitor. There was no harm in Rourke's continuing to try. The doctor increased the Pitocin dose slightly, to as high as the baby's heart rate seemed to allow. Despite the epidural, the contractions became fiercely painful. And there was progress: by 3:00 P.M., Rourke's cervix had dilated to nearly nine centimeters. The contractions had pushed the baby forward two centimeters. Even Peccei began to think Rourke might make this delivery happen.

After three more hours, however, the baby's head was no lower and was still sideways; Rourke's cervix hadn't dilated any further. Rourke finally admitted to herself that her baby wasn't coming out. When Peccei offered her a Cesarean again, she said yes.

The Pitocin drip was turned off. The contraction monitor was removed. There was just the swift tock-tock-tock of the fetal heart monitor. Peccei introduced a colleague who would do the operation—Rourke had been in labor so long, she'd gone through three shifts of obstetricians. She was wheeled to a spacious, white-tiled operating room down the hall. Her husband, Chris, struggled to put on the green scrubs, tie-on mask, bouffant surgical cap, and blue booties over his shoes. He took a chair next to her at the head of the operating table and placed his hand on her shoulder. The anesthesiologist put extra medication in her epidural and pricked at the skin of her belly to make sure that the band of numbness was wide enough. The nurse painted her skin with a yellow-brown antiseptic. Then the cutting began.

The Cesarean section is among the strangest operations I have seen. It is also one of the most straightforward. You press a No. 10 blade down through the flesh, along a side-to-side line low on the bulging abdomen. You divide the skin and golden fat with clean, broad strokes. Using a white gauze pad, you stanch the bleeding points that appear like red blossoms. You slice through the fascia covering the abdominal muscle, a husklike fibrous sheath, and lift it to reveal the beefy red muscle underneath. The rectus abdominis muscle lies in two vertical belts that you part in the middle like a curtain, metal retractors pulling left and right. You cut through the peritoneum, a thin, almost translucent membrane. And the uterus—plum-colored, thick, and muscular—gapes into view. You make a small, initial opening in the uterus with the scalpel, and then you switch to bandage scissors to open it more swiftly and easily. It's as if you're cutting open a tough, leathery fruit.

Then comes what still seems surreal to me. You reach in, and instead of finding a tumor or some other abnormality, as surgeons usually do when we go into someone's belly, you find five tiny wiggling toes, a knee, a whole leg. And suddenly you realize you have a new human being struggling in your hands. You almost forget the mother on the table. The infant can sometimes be hard to get out. If the head is deep in the birth canal, you have to grab around the waist, stand up tall, and *pulllll*. Sometimes you have to have someone push on the baby's head from below. Then the umbilical cord is cut. The baby is swaddled. The nurse records the Apgar score.

After the next uterine contraction, you deliver the placenta through the wound. With a fresh gauze pad, you wipe the inside of the mother's uterus clean of clots and debris. You sew it closed with two baseball-stitched layers of stout absorbable suture. You sew the muscle fascia back together with another suture, then sew the skin. And you are done.

This procedure, once a rarity, is now commonplace. Where before obstetricians learned one technique for a foot dangling out, another for a breech with its arms above its head, yet another for a baby with its head jammed inside the pelvis, all tricky in their own individual ways, now the solution is the same almost regardless of the problem: the C-section. Every obstetrician today is comfortable doing C-sections. Small hospitals have no difficulty keeping in practice. The procedure is performed with impressive consistency.

As straightforward as these operations are, they can go wrong. The child can be lacerated. If the placenta separates and the head doesn't come free quickly, the baby can asphyxiate. The mother faces significant risks, too. As a surgeon, I have been called in to help repair bowel that was torn and wounds that split open. Bleeding can be severe. Wound infections are common. There are increased risks of blood clots and pneumonia. Even without any complication, the recovery is weeks longer and more painful than with vaginal delivery. And, in future pregnancies, mothers can face serious difficulties. The uterine scar has a one in two hundred chance of rupturing in an attempted vaginal delivery. There's a similar risk that the scar could attach itself to a new baby's placenta and cause difficult bleeding problems. C-sections are surgery. There is no getting around it.

Yet there's also no getting around C-sections. We have reached the point that, when there's any question of delivery risk, the Cesarean is what clinicians turn to—it's simply the most reliable option. If a mother is carrying a baby more than ten pounds in size, if she's had a C-section before, if the baby is lying sideways or in a breech position, if she has twins, if any

number of potentially difficult situations for delivery arise—
the standard of care requires that a midwife or an obstetrician
at least offer a Cesarean section. Clinicians are increasingly reluctant to take a risk, however small, and try laboring through.

I asked Bowes how he would have handled obstructed
deliveries like Rourke's back in the sixties. His first recourse, as
you'd expect, would have included the forceps.* He had delivered more than a thousand babies with forceps, he said, with a
rate of neonatal injury as good as or better than with Cesarean sections, and a far faster recovery for the mothers. Had
Rourke been under his care back then, the odds are excellent
that she could have delivered safely without surgery. But
Bowes is a virtuoso of a difficult instrument. When the protocols of his profession changed, he changed with them. "As a
professor, you have to be a role model. You don't want to be
the cowboy who goes in to do something that your residents
are not going to be able to do," he told me. "And there was always uncertainty." Even he had to worry that, someday, his
judgment and skill would fail him.

These were the rules of the factory floor. To discourage
the inexpert from using forceps—along with all those epony-
mous maneuvers—obstetrics had to discourage everyone
from using them. When Bowes finished his career, in 1999, he
had a 24 percent Cesarean rate, just like the rest of his colleagues. He has little doubt he'd be approaching 30 percent,
like his colleagues today, if he were still practicing.

*Earlier in labor, he would have increased the Pitocin dose to far higher
amounts than we accept today, in order to bring her cervix to full dilation. Then
he would have put the forceps on.

A measure of how safe Cesareans have become is that there is a ferocious but genuine debate about whether a mother in the thirty-ninth week of pregnancy with no special risks should be offered a Cesarean delivery as an alternative to wait-ing for labor. The idea seems the worst kind of hubris. How could a Cesarean delivery be considered without even trying a natural one? Surgeons don't suggest that healthy people get their appendixes taken out or that artificial hips might be stronger than the standard-issue ones. Our complication rates for even simple procedures remain unflatteringly high. Yet, in the next decade or so, the industrial revolution in obstetrics could well make Cesarean delivery consistently safer than the birth process that evolution gave us.

Currently, one baby out of five hundred who are healthy and kicking at thirty-nine weeks dies before or during childbirth—a historically low rate, but obstetricians have rea-son to believe that scheduled C-sections could avert at least some of these deaths. Many argue that the results for moth-ers are safe, too. Scheduled C-sections are certainly far less risky than emergency C-sections—procedures done quickly, in dire circumstances, for mothers and babies already in dis-tress. One recent American study has raised concerns about whether scheduled C-sections are safe enough or not, but a study in Britain and one in Israel actually found that sched-uled C-sections had lower maternal mortality than vaginal delivery. Mothers who undergo planned C-sections may also (though this remains largely speculation) have fewer prob-lems later in life with incontinence and uterine prolapse.

Yet there is something disquieting about the idea that

childbirth is becoming so readily surgical. Some hospitals across the country are doing Cesarean sections in more than half of child deliveries. It is not merely nostalgic to find this disturbing. We are losing our connection to yet another natural process of life. And we are seeing the waning of the art of childbirth, too. The skill to bring a child in trouble safely through a vaginal delivery, however inconsistent and unevenly distributed, has been nurtured over centuries. In the obstetrical mainstream, it won't be long before it is lost.

Skeptics have noted that Cesarean delivery is suspiciously convenient for obstetrician's schedules and, hour for hour, is paid more handsomely than vaginal birth. Obstetricians say that fear of malpractice suits pushes them to do C-sections more readily than even they consider necessary. Putting so many mothers through surgery is hardly cause for celebration. But our deep-seated desire to limit risk to babies is the biggest force behind its prevalence; it is the price extracted by the reliability we aspire to.

In a sense, there is a tyranny to the score. While we rate the newborn child's health, the mother's pain and blood loss and length of recovery seem to count for little. We have no score for how the mother does, beyond asking whether she lived or not—no measure to prod us to improve results for her, too. Yet this imbalance, at least, can surely be righted. If the child's well-being can be measured, why not the mother's, too? Indeed, we need an Apgar score for everyone who encounters medicine: the psychiatry patient, the patient on the hospital ward, the person going through an operation, and, yes, the mother in childbirth, as well. My research group recently came up with a surgical Apgar score—a ten-point rating based on the amount of blood loss, the lowest heart rate, and the lowest blood pressure a patient experiences during an operation. Among almost a thousand patients we tested it in, those with a score of nine or ten had a less than 4 percent chance of complications and there were no deaths; those with a score less than five had a greater than 50 percent chance of complications and a 14 percent chance of death. All patients deserve a simple measure that indicates how well or badly they have come through and that pushes the rest of us to innovate. There is no reason we cannot aim for everyone to do better.

"I WATCHED, YOU know," Rourke says. "I could see the whole thing in the surgical lights. I saw her head come out!" Katherine Anne was born seven pounds, fifteen ounces, with brown hair, blue-gray eyes, and soft purple welts where her head had been wedged sideways deep inside her mother's pelvis. Her Apgar score was eight at one minute and nine at five minutes—nearly perfect.

Her mother had a harder time. "I was a wreck," Rourke says. "I was so exhausted I was basically stuporous. And I had unbearable pain." She'd gone through almost forty hours of labor and a Cesarean section. Peccei told her the next morning, "You got whipped two ways, and you are going to be a mess." She was so debilitated that her milk did not come in.

"I felt like a complete failure, like everything I had set out to do I failed to do," Rourke says. "I didn't want the epidural and then I begged for the epidural. I didn't want a C-section, and I consented to a C-section. I wanted to breast-feed the baby, and I utterly failed to breast-feed." She was miserable for a week. "Then one day I realized, 'You know what? This is a stupid thing to think. You have a totally gorgeous little child and it's time to pay a little more attention to your totally gorgeous little child.' Somehow she let me put all my regrets behind me."

The Bell Curve

Finding a meaningful way to measure performance, as Virginia Apgar showed was possible in child delivery, is a form of ingenuity in itself. What you actually do with that measure involves another type of ingenuity, however, and improvement ultimately requires both kinds. One person who has understood this is a Minneapolis doctor who has spent four decades perfecting care for a single, rare, and fatal disease. His experience holds a lesson for all of us. In order to tell you his story, though, I need to first tell you about Annie Page, a young girl who was discovered to have the disease.

Annie Page's illness began with the kinds of small, unexceptional details that mean nothing until seen in hindsight. Like the fact that, when she was a baby, her father sometimes called her Little Potato Chip, because her skin tasted salty when he kissed her. Or that Annie's mother noticed that her breathing was sometimes a little wheezy, though the pediatrician heard nothing through his stethoscope.

The detail that finally mattered was Annie's size. For a while, Annie's fine-boned petiteness seemed to be just a family trait. Her sister, Lauryn, four years older, had always been at the bottom end of the pediatrician's growth chart for girls her age. By the time Annie was three years old, however, she had fallen off the chart. She stood an acceptable thirty-four inches tall but weighed only twenty-three pounds—less than 98 percent of girls her age. She did not look malnourished, but she didn't look quite healthy, either.

"Failure to thrive" is what it's called, and there can be scores of explanations: pituitary disorders, hypothyroidism, genetic defects in metabolism, inflammatory-bowel disease, lead poisoning, HIV, tapeworm infection. In textbooks, the complete list is at least a page long. Annie's doctor did a thorough workup. Then, at four o'clock on July 27, 1997— "I'll never forget that day," her mother, Honor, says—the pediatrician called the Pages at home with the results of a sweat test.

It's a funny little test. The skin on the inside surface of a child's forearm is cleaned and dried. Two small gauze pads are applied—one soaked with pilocarpine, a medicine that makes skin sweat, and the other with a salt solution. Electrodes are hooked up. Then a mild electric current is turned on for five minutes, driving the pilocarpine into the skin. A reddened, sweaty area about an inch in diameter appears on the skin, and a collection pad of dry filter paper is taped over it to absorb the sweat for half an hour. A technician then measures the concentration of chloride in the pad.

Over the phone, the doctor told Honor that her daughter's chloride level was far higher than normal. Honor is a hospital pharmacist, and she had come across children with abnormal results like this. "All I knew was that it meant she was going to die," she said quietly when I visited the Pages' home, in the Cincinnati suburb of Loveland. The test showed that Annie had cystic fibrosis.

Cystic fibrosis is a genetic disease. Only a thousand American children per year are diagnosed as having it. Some ten million people in the United States carry the defective gene, but the disorder is recessive: a child will develop the condition only if both parents are carriers and both pass on a copy. The gene—which was discovered, in 1989, sitting out on the long arm of chromosome No. 7—produces a mutant protein that interferes with cells' ability to manage chloride. This is what makes sweat from people with CF so salty. (Salt is sodium chloride, after all.) The chloride defect thickens secretions throughout the body, turning them dry and gluey. In the ducts of the pancreas, the flow of digestive enzymes becomes blocked, making a child less and less able to absorb food. This was the reason Annie had all but stopped growing. The effects on the lungs, however, are what make the disease lethal. Thickened mucus slowly fills the small airways and hardens, shrinking lung capacity. Over time, the disease leaves a child with the equivalent of just one functioning lung. Then half a lung. Then none at all.

The one overwhelming thought in the minds of Honor and Don Page was: We need to get to Children's. Cincinnati Children's Hospital is among the most respected pediatric hospitals in the country. It was where Albert Sabin invented the oral polio vaccine. The chapter on cystic fibrosis in the *Nelson Textbook of Pediatrics*—the bible of the specialty—was written by one of the hospital's pediatricians. The Pages called and were given an appointment for the next morning.

"We were there for hours, meeting with all the different members of the team," Honor recalled. "They took Annie's blood pressure, measured her oxygen saturation, did some other tests. Then they put us in a room, and the pediatrician sat down with us. He was very kind, but frank, too. He said, 'Do you understand it's a genetic disease? That it's nothing you did, nothing you can catch?' He told us the median survival for patients was thirty years. In Annie's lifetime, he said, we could see that go to forty. For him, he was sharing a great accomplishment in CF care. And the news was better than our worst fears. But only forty! That's not what we wanted to hear."

The team members reviewed the treatments. The Pages were told that they would have to give Annie pancreatic-enzyme pills with the first bite of every meal. They would have to give her supplemental vitamins. They also had to add calories wherever they could—putting tablespoons of butter on everything, giving her ice cream whenever she wanted, and then putting chocolate sauce on it.

A respiratory therapist explained that they would need to do manual chest therapy at least twice a day, half-hour sessions in which they would strike—"percuss"—their daughter's torso with a cupped hand at each of fourteen specific locations on the front, back, and sides in order to loosen the thick secretions and help her to cough them up. They were given prescriptions for inhaled medicines. The doctor told them that Annie would need to come back once every three months for extended checkups. And then they went home to start their new life. They had been told almost everything they needed to know in order to give Annie her best chance to live as long as possible.

The one thing that the clinicians failed to tell them, however, was that Cincinnati Children's was not, as the Pages supposed, among the country's top centers for children with cystic fibrosis. According to data from that year, it was, at best, an average program. This was no small matter. In 1997, patients at an average center were living to be just over thirty years old; patients at the top center typically lived to be forty-six. By some measures, Cincinnati was well below average. The best predictor of a CF patient's life expectancy is his or her lung function. At Cincinnati, the lung function achieved by patients under the age of twelve—children like Annie—remained in the bottom 25 percent of the country's CF patients. And the doctors there knew it.

IT USED TO be assumed that differences among hospitals or doctors in a particular specialty were generally insignificant. If you plotted a graph showing the results of all the centers treating cystic fibrosis—or any other disease, for that matter—people expected that the curve would look something like a shark fin:

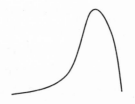

with most places clustered around the very best outcomes. But the evidence has begun to indicate otherwise. What you tend to find instead is a bell curve:

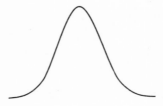

with a handful of teams showing disturbingly poor outcomes for their patients, a handful obtaining remarkably good results, and a great undistinguished middle.

After an ordinary hernia operation, for example, the chances a patient will have a recurrent hernia are one in ten with surgeons at the unhappy end of the spectrum, one in twenty with those in the middle majority, and under one in five hundred with an elite handful. For newborns admitted to a neonatal intensive care unit, the risk-adjusted death rate averages 10 percent but varies from 6 to 16 percent, depending on the center. For women undergoing in vitro fertilization, the likelihood of successful pregnancy from a given attempt at implanting a fertilized embryo is around 40 percent for most centers but ranges from under 15 percent to over 65 percent depending on where they go. Differences in the age of patients a center sees, its willingness to accept high-risk patients, and other factors certainly account for some of this variability. Nonetheless, for a given patient, there are wide, meaningful differences among centers and a few are simply better than the rest.

The bell curve is distressing for doctors to have to acknowledge. It belies the promise that we make to patients: that they can count on the medical system to give them their very best chance. It also contradicts the belief nearly all of us have that we are doing our job as well as it can be done. But evidence of the bell curve is starting to trickle out, to doctors and patients alike, and we are only beginning to find out what happens when it does.

In medicine, we are used to confronting failure; all doctors have unforeseen deaths and complications. What we're not used to doing is comparing our records of success and failure with those of our peers. I am a surgeon in a department that is, our members like to believe, one of the best in the country. But the truth is that we have had no reliable evidence about whether we're as good as we think we are. Baseball teams have win-loss records. Businesses have quarterly earnings reports. What about doctors?

There is a company on the Web called HealthGrades, which for $17.95 will give you a report card on any physician you choose. Not long ago, I requested the company's report cards on me and several of my colleagues. They don't tell you that much. You will learn, for instance, that I am certified in my specialty, have no criminal convictions, have not been fired from any hospital, have not had my license suspended or revoked, and have not been disciplined for misconduct. This is no doubt useful to know. But it sets the bar a tad low, doesn't it?

In recent years, there has been a proliferation of efforts to measure how various hospitals and doctors perform. No one has found the task easy. One difficulty has been figuring out what to measure. For six years, from 1986 to 1992, the federal government released an annual report that came to be known as the Death List. It ranked all the hospitals in the country by their death rate for elderly and disabled patients on Medicare. The spread was alarmingly wide, and the Death List made headlines the first year it came out. But the rankings proved to be almost useless. Death among the elderly or disabled mostly has to do with how old or sick they are to begin with, and the statisticians could never quite work out how to apportion blame between nature and doctors. Volatility in the numbers was one sign of the trouble. Hospitals' rankings seesawed dramatically from one year to the next due to a handful of random deaths. It was unclear what kind of changes would improve their performance (other than sending their sickest patients to other hospitals). Pretty soon the public simply ignored the rankings.

Even with younger patients, death rates are a poor metric for how doctors do. After all, very few young patients die, and when they do it's rarely a surprise; most already have metastatic cancer or horrendous injuries or the like. What one really wants to know is how we perform in typical circumstances—some kind of score for the immediate results, perhaps, and also a measure of the processes involved. For patients with pneumonia, how often does my hospital get them the correct antibiotic, and on the whole how do they do? How do our results compare with those of other hospitals?

Gathering this kind of data can be difficult. Medicine still relies heavily on paper records, so to collect information you have to send people to either scour the charts or track the patients themselves, both of which are expensive and laborious propositions. Recent privacy regulations have made the task still harder. Yet it is starting to be done. The country's veterans' hospitals have all now brought in staff who do nothing but record and compare surgeons' complication rates and death rates. Fourteen teaching hospitals, including my own, have recently joined together to do the same. California, New Jersey, New York, and Pennsylvania have been collecting and reporting data on every cardiac surgeon in their states for years.

ONE SMALL FIELD in medicine has been far ahead of most others in measuring the results its practitioners achieve: cystic fibrosis care. For forty years, the Cystic Fibrosis Foundation has gathered detailed data from the country's cystic fibrosis treatment centers. It did so not because it is more enlightened than everyone else but because, in the 1960s, a pediatrician from Cleveland named LeRoy Matthews was driving people in the field crazy.

Matthews had started a cystic fibrosis treatment program as a young pulmonary specialist at Babies and Children's Hospital in Cleveland, in 1957, and within a few years was claiming to have an annual mortality rate of less than 2 percent. To anyone treating CF at the time, it was a preposterous assertion. National mortality rates for the disease were estimated to be higher than 20 percent a year, and the average patient died by the age of three. Yet here was Matthews saying that he and his colleagues could stop the disease from doing serious harm for years. "How long [our patients] will live remains to be seen, but I expect most of them to come to my funeral," he told one conference of physicians.

In 1964, the Cystic Fibrosis Foundation gave a University

of Minnesota pediatrician named Warren Warwick a modest budget of ten thousand dollars to collect reports on every patient treated at the thirty-one CF centers in the United States that year—data that would test Matthews's claim. Several months later, he had the results: the median estimated age at death for patients in Matthews's center was twenty-one years, seven times the age of patients treated elsewhere. Matthews was what we'd now call a positive deviant. He had not had a single death among patients younger than six in at least five years.

Unlike pediatricians elsewhere, Matthews viewed CF not as a sudden affliction but as a cumulative disease and provided aggressive preventive treatment to stave it off long before his patients became visibly sick from it. He made his patients sleep each night in a plastic tent filled with a continuous aerosolized water mist so dense you could barely see through it. This thinned the tenacious mucus that clogged their airways, enabling them to cough it up. Using an innovation of British pediatricians, he also had family members clap on the children's chests daily to help loosen the mucus. After Warwick's report came out, Matthews's treatment quickly became the standard in this country. The American Thoracic Society endorsed his approach, and Warwick's data registry on treatment centers proved so useful that the Cystic Fibrosis Foundation has continued it ever since.

Looking at the data over time is both fascinating and disconcerting. By 1966, mortality from CF nationally had dropped so much that the average life expectancy of CF patients had already reached ten years. By 1972, it was eighteen years—a rapid and remarkable transformation. At the same time, though, Matthews's center had got even better. The foundation never identified individual centers in its data; to ensure participation, it guaranteed anonymity. But Matthews's center published its results. By the early 1970s, 95 percent of patients who had gone there before severe lung disease set in were living past their eighteenth birthday. There was a bell curve, and the spread had narrowed a little. Yet every time the average moved up, Matthews and a few others somehow managed to stay ahead of the pack.

In 2003, life expectancy with CF had risen to thirty-three years nationally, but at the best center it was more than forty-seven. Experts have become as leery of life-expectancy calculations as they are of hospital death rates, but other measures tell the same story. For example, at the median center, lung function for patients with CF—the best predictor of survival—is about three-quarters of what it is for people without CF. At the top centers, the average lung function of patients is indistinguishable from that of children who do not have CF. Some allege that the differences are explained simply by the differences in the specific gene patients inherit or by the social class of their families. But according to a recent study, such factors, even taken together, explain at best a quarter of the variability—and nothing about how some centers have kept their average CF patient as normal as children without the disease.

What makes the wide variability especially puzzling is that our system for CF care is so much more sophisticated than that for most other diseases. CF care works the way we want all of medicine to work. Patients receive care in one of 117 ultraspecialized centers across the country. All centers undergo a rigorous certification process. Their doctors have a high volume of experience in caring for people with CF. They all follow the same guidelines for CF treatment, guidelines that are far more detailed than we have in most of medicine. They all participate in research trials to figure out new and better treatments. You would think, therefore, that their results would be much the same. Yet the differences are enormous. Patients have not known this. So what happens when they find out?

IN THE WINTER of 2001, the Pages and twenty other families were invited by their doctors at Cincinnati Children's to a meeting about the CF program there. Annie was seven years old now, a lively second grader. She was still not growing enough, and a simple cold could be hellish for her, but her lung function had been stable. The families gathered in a large conference room at the hospital. After a brief introduction, the doctors started flashing PowerPoint slides on a screen: here is how the top programs do on nutrition and respiratory performance, and here is how Cincinnati does. It was a kind of experiment in openness. The doctors were nervous. Some were opposed to having the meeting at all. But hospital leaders had insisted on going ahead. The reason was Don Berwick.

Berwick is a former pediatrician who runs a nonprofit organization in Boston called the Institute for Healthcare Improvement. The institute has provided multimillion-dollar grants to hospitals that are willing to try his ideas for improving medical practice. Cincinnati's CF program won one of the grants. And among Berwick's key stipulations was that recipients had to open up their information to their patients—to "go naked," as one doctor put it.

Berwick is an unusual figure in medicine. In 2002, the industry publication *Modern Healthcare* listed him as the third most powerful person in American health care. Unlike the others on the list, he is powerful not because of the position he holds. (The secretary of health and human services was No. 1, and the head of Medicare and Medicaid was No. 2.) He is powerful because of how he thinks.

At a conference in December 1999, Berwick gave a forty-minute speech distilling his ideas about the failings of American health care. Years afterward, people are still talking about the speech. The video of it circulated like samizdat. (That was how I saw it—on a grainy, overplayed VHS tape—about a year later.) A booklet with the transcript was sent to thousands of doctors around the country. Berwick is middle-aged, soft-spoken, and unprepossessing, and he knows how to use his apparent ordinariness to his advantage. He began his speech with a gripping story about a 1949 Montana forest fire that engulfed a parachute brigade of firefighters. Panicking, they ran, trying to make it up a 76 percent grade and over a crest to safety. But their commander, a man named Wag Dodge, saw that their plan wasn't going to work. So he stopped, took out some matches, and set the tall dry grass ahead of him on fire. The new blaze caught and rapidly spread up the slope. He stepped into the middle of the burned-out area it left behind, lay down, and called out to his crew to join him. He had invented, on the spot, what came to be called an "escape fire," and it later became a standard part of Forest Service fire training.

His men, however, either thought he was crazy or never heard his calls, and they ran past him. All but two were caught by the inferno and perished. Inside his escape fire, Dodge survived virtually unharmed.

As Berwick explained, the firefighters' organization had unraveled. The men had lost their ability to think coherently, to act together, to recognize that a lifesaving idea might be possible. This is what happens to all flawed organizations in a disaster, and, he argued, this is what is happening in modern health care. As medicine tries to cope with the advancing complexity of knowledge and treatment, it is falling short in performing even the simplest of its tasks. To fix medicine, Berwick maintained, we need to do two things: measure ourselves and be more open about what we are doing. We should be routinely comparing the performance of doctors and hospitals, looking at everything from surgical complication rates to how often a drug ordered for a patient is delivered correctly and on time. And, he insisted, hospitals should give patients total access to the information. " 'No secrets' is the new rule in my escape fire," he said. He argued that openness would drive improvement, if simply through embarrassment. It would make it clear that the well-being and convenience of patients, not of doctors, were paramount. It would also serve a fundamental moral good, because people should be able to learn about anything that affects their lives.

Berwick's institute was given serious money from the Robert Wood Johnson Foundation to offer to those who used his ideas. And so the doctors, nurses, and social workers of Cincinnati Children's stood uncertainly before a crowd of patients' families in that hospital conference room, told them how poorly the program's results ranked, and announced a plan for doing better. Surprisingly, not a single family chose to leave the program.

"We thought about it after that meeting," Ralph Blackwelder told me. He and his wife, Tracey, have eight children, four of whom have CF. "We thought maybe we should move. We could sell my business here and start a business somewhere else. We were thinking, Why would I want my kids to be seen here, with inferior care? I want the very best people to be helping my children." But he and Tracey were impressed that the team had told them the truth. No one at Cincinnati Children's had made any excuses, and everyone appeared desperate to do better. The Blackwelders had known these people for years. The program's nutritionist, Terri Schindler, had a child of her own in the program. Their pulmonary specialist, Barbara Chini, had been smart, attentive, and loving—taking their late-night phone calls, seeing the children through terrible crises, instituting new therapies as they became available. The program director, Jim Acton, made a personal promise that there would soon be no better treatment center in the world.

Honor Page was alarmed when she saw the numbers. Like the Blackwelders, the Pages had a close relationship with the team at Children's, but the news tested their loyalty. Acton announced the formation of several committees that would work to improve the program's results. Each committee, he said, had to have at least one parent on it. This is unusual; hospitals seldom allow patients and families on internal-review committees. So, rather than walk away, Honor decided to sign up for the committee that would reexamine the science behind patients' care.

Her committee was puzzled that the center's results were not better. Not only had the center followed national guidelines for CF, but two of its physicians had helped write them. The committee wanted to visit the top centers, but no one knew which those were. Although the Cystic Fibrosis Foundation's annual reports displayed the individual results for each of the country's 117 centers, no names were attached. Doctors put in a call and sent e-mails to the foundation, asking for the names of the top five, but to no avail.

Several months later, in early 2002, Don Berwick visited the Cincinnati program. He was impressed by its sincere desire to improve and by the intense involvement of the families, but he was incredulous when he learned that the committee couldn't get the names of the top programs from the foundation. He called the foundation's executive vice president for medical affairs, Preston Campbell, who reacted with instinctive caution. The centers, he tried to explain, give their data voluntarily. The reason they have done so for forty years is that they have trusted that the data would be kept confidential. Once the centers lose that faith, they might no longer report solid information tracking how different treatments are working, and how well they do.

Campbell is a deliberate and thoughtful man, a pediatric pulmonologist who has devoted his career to cystic fibrosis patients. The discussion with Berwick had left him uneasy. The Cystic Fibrosis Foundation had always been dedicated to the value of research; by investing in bench science, it had helped decode the gene for cystic fibrosis, produce two new drugs approved for patients, and generate more than a dozen other drugs that are currently being tested. Its investments in tracking patient care had resulted in scores of valuable studies that had resulted in new guidelines, tighter standards for certification, more regularized care. Yet their research also showed that patients continued to get care of widely differing quality.

A couple of weeks after Berwick's phone call, Campbell released the names of the top five centers to Cincinnati. Indeed, he'd become himself persuaded that further improvement would come only through greater transparency. In 2004, the foundation announced a goal of eventually making the outcomes of every center publicly available. But, it insisted, it needed time to achieve this. Only a few of the nation's CF treatment centers had actually agreed to go public.

Still, after traveling to one of the top five centers for a look, I found I could not avoid naming the center I saw—no obscuring physicians' identities or glossing over details. There was simply no way to explain what a great center did without the particulars. The people from Cincinnati found this, too. Within months of learning which the top five centers were, they'd spoken to people at each and then visited what they considered to be the very best one, the Minnesota Cystic Fibrosis Center, at Fairview-University Children's Hospital, in Minneapolis. I went first to Cincinnati and then to Minneapolis for comparison.

What I saw in Cincinnati both impressed me and, given its middling ranking, surprised me. The members of the CF staff were skilled, energetic, and dedicated. They had just completed a flu-vaccination campaign that had reached more than 90 percent of their patients. Before clinic visits, patients filled out questionnaires so that the team would be better prepared for the questions they would have and the services (such as X-rays, tests, and specialist consultations) they would need. Before patients went home, the doctors gave them a written summary of their visit and a complete copy of their record, something that I had never thought to do in my own practice.

I joined Cori Daines, one of the seven CF care specialists, in her clinic one morning. Among the patients we saw was Alyssa. She was fifteen years old, freckled, skinny, with nails painted loud red, straight sandy blond hair tied in a ponytail, a soda in one hand, legs crossed, foot bouncing constantly. Every few minutes, she gave a short, throaty cough. Her parents sat to one side. All the questions were directed to her. How had she been doing? How was school going? Any breathing difficulties? Trouble keeping up with her calories? Her answers were monosyllabic at first. But Daines had known Alyssa for years, and slowly she opened up. Things had mostly been going all right, she said. She had been sticking with her treatment regimen—twice-a-day manual chest therapy by one of her parents, inhaled medications using a nebulizer immediately afterward, and vitamins. Her lung function had been measured that morning, and it was 67 percent of normal—slightly down from her usual 80 percent. Her cough had got a little worse the day before, and this was thought to be the reason for the dip. Daines was concerned about stomach pains that Alyssa had been having for several months. The pains came on unpredictably, Alyssa said—before meals, after meals, in the middle of the night. They were sharp and persisted for up to a couple of hours. Examinations, tests, and X-rays had found no abnormalities, but she'd stayed home from school for the past five weeks. Her parents, exasperated because she seemed fine most of the time, wondered if the pain could be just in her head. Daines wasn't sure. She asked a staff nurse to check in with Alyssa at home, arranged for a consultation with a gastroenterologist and with a pain specialist, and scheduled an earlier return visit than the usual three months.

This was, it seemed to me, real medicine: untidy, human, but practiced carefully and conscientiously—as well as anyone could ask for. Then I went to Minneapolis.

THE DIRECTOR OF Fairview-University Children's Hospital's cystic fibrosis center for almost forty years has been none other than Warren Warwick, the pediatrician who had conducted the study of LeRoy Matthews's suspiciously high success rate. Ever since then, Warwick has made a study of what it takes to do better than everyone else. The secret, he insists, is simple, and he learned it from Matthews: you do whatever you can to keep your patients' lungs as open as possible. Patients with CF at Fairview got the same things that patients everywhere got—some nebulized treatments to loosen secretions and unclog passageways (a kind of mist tent in a mouth pipe), antibiotics, and a good thumping on their chests every day. Yet, somehow, everything Warwick did was different.

In the clinic one afternoon, I joined him as he saw a seventeen-year-old high school senior named Janelle, who had been diagnosed with CF at the age of six and had been under his care ever since. She had come for her routine three-month checkup. She wore dyed black hair to her shoulder blades, black Avril Lavigne eyeliner, four earrings in each ear, two more in an eyebrow, and a stud in her tongue. Warwick was seventy-six years old, tall, stooped, and frumpy-looking, with a well-worn tweed jacket, liver spots dotting his skin, wispy gray hair—by all appearances, a doddering, midcentury academic. He stood in front of Janelle for a moment, hands on his hips, looking her over, and then he said, "So, Janelle, what have you been doing to make us the best CF program in the country?"

"It's not easy, you know," she said.

They bantered. She was doing fine. School was going well. Warwick pulled out her latest lung-function measurements. There'd been a slight dip, as there was with Alyssa. Three months earlier, Janelle had been at 109 percent (she was actually doing better than the average child without CF); now she was at around 90 percent. That was still pretty good, and some ups and downs in the numbers are to be expected. But this was not the way Warwick saw the results.

He knitted his eyebrows. "Why did they go down?" he asked.

Janelle shrugged.

Any cough lately? No. Colds? No. Fevers? No. Was she sure she'd been taking her treatments regularly? Yes, of course. Every day? Yes. Did she ever miss treatments? Sure. Everyone does once in a while. How often is once in a while?

Then, slowly, Warwick got a different story out of her: in the past few months, it turned out, she'd barely been taking her treatments at all.

He pressed on. "Why aren't you taking your treatments?" He appeared neither surprised nor angry. He seemed genuinely curious, as if he'd never run across this interesting situation before.

"I don't know."

He kept pushing. "What keeps you from doing your treatments?"

"I don't know."

"Up here"—he pointed at his own head—"what's going on?"

"*I. Don't. Know,*" she said.

He paused for a moment. Then he turned to me, taking a new tack. "The thing about patients with CF is that they're good scientists," he said. "They always experiment. We have to help them interpret what they experience as they experiment. So they stop doing their treatments. And what happens? They don't get sick. Therefore, they conclude, Dr. Warwick is nuts."

"But let's look at the numbers," he said to me, ignoring Janelle. He went to a little blackboard he had on the wall. It appeared to be well used. "A person's daily risk of getting a bad lung illness with CF is 0.5 percent." He wrote the number down. Janelle rolled her eyes. She began tapping her foot. "The daily risk of getting a bad lung illness with CF plus treatment is 0.05 percent," he went on, and he wrote that number down. "So when you experiment you're looking at the difference between a 99.5 percent chance of staying well and a 99.95 percent chance of staying well. Seems hardly any difference, right? On any given day, you have basically a one-hundred-percent chance of being well. But"—he paused and took a step toward me—"it is a big difference." He chalked out the calculations.

"Sum it up over a year, and it is the difference between an 83 percent chance of making it through [the year] without getting sick and only a 16 percent chance."

He turned to Janelle. "How do you stay well all your life? How do you become a geriatric patient?" he asked her. Her foot finally stopped tapping. "I can't promise you anything. I can only tell you the odds."

In this short speech, I realized, was the core of Warwick's worldview. He believed that excellence came from seeing, on a daily basis, the difference between being 99.5 percent successful and being 99.95 percent successful. Many things human beings do are like that, of course: catching fly balls, manufacturing microchips, delivering overnight packages. Medicine's distinction is that lives are lost in those slim margins.

And so he went to work on finding that margin for Janelle. Eventually, he figured out that she had a new boyfriend. She had a new job, too, and was working nights. The boyfriend had his own apartment, and she was either there or at a friend's house most of the time, so she rarely made it home to take her treatments. At school, new rules required her to go to the nurse for each dose of medicine during the day. So she skipped going. "It's such a pain," she said. He learned that there were some medicines she took and some she didn't. One she took because it was the only thing that she felt actually made a difference. She took her vitamins, too. ("Why your vitamins?" "Because they're cool.") The rest she ignored.

Warwick proposed a deal. Janelle would go home for a breathing treatment every day after school and get her best friend to hold her to it. She'd also keep key medications in her bag or her pocket at school and take them on her own. ("The nurse won't let me." "Don't tell her," he said, and deftly turned taking care of herself into an act of rebellion.) So far, Janelle was OK with this. But there was one other thing, he said: she'd have to come to the hospital for a few days of therapy to recover the lost ground. She stared at him.

"Today?"

"Yes, today."

"How about tomorrow?"

"We've failed, Janelle," he said. "It's important to acknowledge when we've failed."

With that, she began to cry.

WARWICK'S COMBINATION OF focus, aggressiveness, and inventiveness is what makes him extraordinary. He thinks hard about his patients, he pushes them, and he does not hesitate to improvise. Twenty years ago, while he was listening to a church choir and mulling over how he might examine his patients better, he came up with a new stethoscope—a stereo-stethoscope, he calls it. It has two bells dangling from it and, because of a built-in sound delay, transmits lung sounds in stereo. He had an engineer make it for him. Listening to Janelle with the instrument, he put one bell on the right side of her chest and the other on her left side and insisted that he could systematically localize how individual lobes of her lungs sounded.

He invented a new cough. It wasn't enough that his patients actively cough up their sputum. He wanted a deeper, better cough, and later, in his office, Warwick made another patient practice his cough. The patient stretched his arms upward, yawned, pinched his nose, bent down as far as he could, let the pressure build up, and then, straightening, blasted everything out. ("Again!" Warwick encouraged him. "Harder!")

He produced his most far-reaching invention almost two decades ago—a mechanized chest-thumping vest for patients to wear. The chief difficulty for people with CF is sticking with the laborious daily regimen of care, particularly the manual chest therapy. It requires another person's help. It requires conscientiousness, making sure to bang on each of the fourteen locations on the patient's chest. And it requires consistency, doing this twice a day, every day, year after year. Warwick had become fascinated by studies showing that inflating and deflating a blood-pressure cuff around a dog's chest could mobilize its lung secretions, and in the mid-1980s he created what is now known as the Vest. It looks like a black flak jacket with two vacuum hoses coming out of the sides. These are hooked up to a compressor that shoots quick blasts of air in and out of the vest at high frequencies. (I talked to a patient while he had one of these on. He vibrated like a car on a rutted back road.) Studies eventually showed that Warwick's device was at least as effective as manual chest therapy—and was used far more consistently. Today, 45,000 patients with CF and other lung diseases use the technology.

Like most other medical clinics, the Minnesota Cystic Fibrosis Center has several physicians and many more staff members. Warwick established a weekly meeting to review everyone's care for their patients, and he insists on a degree of uniformity that clinicians usually find intolerable. Some chafe. He can have, as one of the doctors put it, "somewhat of an absence of, um, collegial respect for different care plans." And although he stepped down as director of the center in 1999, to let a protégé, Carlos Milla, take over, he remains its guiding spirit. He and his colleagues aren't content if their patients' lung function is 80 percent of normal, or even 90 percent. They aim for 100 percent—or better. Almost 10 percent of the children at his center get supplemental feedings through a latex tube surgically inserted into their stomachs, simply because, by Warwick's standards, they were not gaining enough weight. There's no published research showing that you need to do this. But not a single child or teenager at the center has died in almost a decade. Its oldest patient is now sixty-seven.

In medicine, we have learned to appreciate the danger of ad hoc experimentation on patients—of cowboy physicians. We endeavor to stick to established findings. But with his unblinking focus on his patients' actual results, Warwick has been able to innovate successfully. And he has become almost contemptuous of established findings. National clinical guidelines for care are, he says, "a record of the past, and little more—they should have an expiration date." I accompanied him as he visited another of his patients, Scott Pieper. When Pieper came to Fairview, at the age of thirty-two, he had lost at least 80 percent of his lung capacity. He was too weak and short of breath to take a walk, let alone work, and he wasn't expected to last a year. That was fourteen years ago.

"Some days, I think, This is it—I'm not going to make it," Pieper told me. "But other times I think, I'm going to make sixty, seventy, maybe more." For the past several months, Warwick had Pieper trying a new idea—wearing his vest not only for two daily thirty-minute sessions but also while napping for two hours in the middle of the day. Falling asleep in that shuddering thing took some getting used to. But Pieper was soon able to take up bowling, his first regular activity in years. He joined a two-night-a-week league. He couldn't go four games, and his score always dropped in the third game, but he'd worked his average up to 177. "Any ideas about what we could do so you could last for that extra game, Scott?" Warwick asked. Well, Pieper said, he'd noticed that in the cold—anything below fifty degrees—and when humidity was below 50 percent, he did better. Warwick suggested doing an extra hour in the vest on warm or humid days and on every game day. Pieper said he'd try it.

We are used to thinking that a doctor's ability depends mainly on science and skill. The lesson from Minneapolis—and indeed from battlefield medical tents in Iraq, villages with outbreaks of polio, birthing rooms across the country, and all the other places I have described in this book—is that these may be the easiest parts of care. Even doctors with great knowledge and technical skill can have mediocre results; more nebulous factors like aggressiveness and diligence and ingenuity can matter enormously. In Cincinnati and in Minneapolis, the doctors are equally capable and well versed in the data on CF. But if Annie Page—who has had no breathing problems or major setbacks—were in Minneapolis she would almost certainly have had a feeding tube in her stomach and Warwick's team hounding her to figure out ways to make her breathing even better than normal.

Don Berwick believes that the subtleties of high-performance medical practice can be identified and learned. But the lessons are hidden because no one knows who the high performers really are. Only if we know the results from all can we identify the positive deviants and learn from them. If we are genuinely curious about how the best achieve their results, Berwick believes, then the ideas will spread.

The test of Berwick's theory is now under way. In December 2006, the Cystic Fibrosis Foundation succeeded in persuading its centers to make public their individual results, adjusted for the severity of disease in their populations. The information is now posted for all to see on the foundation Web site, www.cff.org—the first field in medicine to voluntarily do such a thing.

The Cincinnati CF team has already begun monitoring the nutrition and lung function of individual patients the way Warwick does, and it is getting more aggressive about pushing the results higher, too. Yet you have to wonder whether it is possible to replicate people like Warwick, with their intense drive and constant experimenting. In the few years since the Cystic Fibrosis Foundation began bringing together centers willing to share their data, certain patterns have begun to emerge, according to Bruce Marshall, the head of quality improvement for the foundation. All the centers appear to have made significant progress. None, however, have progressed more than centers like Fairview.

"You look at the rates of improvement in different quartiles, and it's the centers in the top quartile that are improving fastest," Marshall says. "They are at risk of breaking away." What the best may have, above all, is a capacity to learn and change—and to do so faster than everyone else.

*   *   *

ONCE WE ACKNOWLEDGE that, no matter how much we improve our average, the bell curve isn't going away, we're left with all sorts of questions. Will being in the bottom half be used against doctors? Will we be expected to tell our patients how we score? Will patients leave us? Will those at the bottom be paid less than those at the top? The answer to all these questions is likely yes.

Recently, for example, there has been a rapid shift toward "paying for quality." (No one ever says "docking for mediocrity," but it amounts to the same thing.) Across the country, insurers like Medicare, Aetna, and the Blue Cross–Blue Shield companies now hold back 10 percent or more of payments to physicians until specific quality goals are met. Medicare has decided not to pay surgeons for intestinal transplantation operations at all unless the doctors achieve a predefined success rate—and it may extend the practice to other procedures. Not surprisingly, this makes doctors anxious. I once sat in on a presentation of the concept to an audience of doctors hearing about it for the first time. By the end, some in the crowd were practically shouting with indignation: We're going to be paid according to our grades? Who is doing the grading? For God's sake, how?

We in medicine are not the only ones being graded nowadays. Firefighters, CEOs, and salesmen are. Even teachers are being graded, and, in some places, being paid accordingly. Yet we all feel uneasy about being judged by such grades. They never seem to measure the right things. They don't take into account circumstances beyond our control.

They are misused; they are unfair. Still, the simple facts remain: there is a bell curve in all human activities, and the differences you measure usually matter.

I asked Honor Page what she would do if, after all her efforts and the efforts of the doctors and nurses at Cincinnati Children's Hospital to ensure that "there was no place better in the world" to receive cystic fibrosis care, the program's comparative performance still rated as resoundingly average.

"I can't believe that's possible," she told me. The staff have worked so hard, she said, that she could not imagine they would fail.

After I pressed her, though, she told me, "I don't think I'd settle for Cincinnati if it remains just average." Then she thought about it some more. Would she really move Annie away from people who had been so devoted all these years, just because of the numbers? Well, maybe. But, at the same time, she wanted me to understand that their effort counted for more than she was able to express.

I do not have to consider these matters for very long before I start thinking about where I would stand on a bell curve for the operations I do. In my area of specialization, surgery for endocrine tumors, I would hope that my statistics prove to be better than those of surgeons who only occasionally do this kind of surgery. But am I up in Warwickian territory? Do I have to answer this question?

The hardest question for anyone who takes responsibility for what he or she does is, What if I turn out to be average? If we took all the surgeons at my level of experience, compared our results, and discovered that I am one of the worst, the answer would be easy: I'd turn in my scalpel. But what if I were a B–? Working as I do in a city that's mobbed with surgeons, how could I justify putting patients under the knife? I could tell myself, Someone's got to be average. If the bell curve is a fact, then so is the reality that most doctors are going to be average. There is no shame in being one of them, right?

Except, of course, there is. What is troubling is not just being average but settling for it. Everyone knows that averageness is, for most of us, our fate. And in certain matters—looks, money, tennis—we would do well to accept this. But in your surgeon, your child's pediatrician, your police department, your local high school? When the stakes are our lives and the lives of our children, we want no one to settle for average.

For Performance

I was in the operating room doing surgery one day, and across the drapes on the anesthesia team was Dr. Mark Simon, a twenty-nine-year-old resident. This was not a difficult case. So we got to talking. I mentioned the cystic fibrosis programs I'd been thinking about, and it turned out the discussion hit closer to home than I'd realized—because Mark has cystic fibrosis. I'd had no idea, although we'd been in on many cases together and he has the short stature and raspy cough one often sees in people with the disease. The illness has been a tremendous struggle, he told me. He managed to stay healthy through his first three years in medical school. But, in his fourth year, his disease progressed, and he had to be hospitalized for four weeks. The next year, in Boston, in residency, he had to miss six weeks. Now, only halfway through his second year, he'd already been hospitalized another month more. He has become, at twenty-nine, all too aware that the average life expectancy for a person with CF is just thirty-three years. So the question we got talking about was: What is more likely to save his life—investment in laboratory science or in efforts to improve how existing medical care performs?

The answer most people would come to is investment in laboratory science—the search for a cure. And in 1989, when scientists discovered the gene for cystic fibrosis, that would have seemed a wise choice: a cure was believed to be only a few years away. Dramatic progress, however, did not occur. Mark has not let go of the hope that a cure will be found. But he was not putting any bets on that happening in time to help him. Instead, he said, his hopes were focused on efforts to monitor and improve and transform clinical performance using know-how already in existence. He believed that of all the work being done, this was the work that would save more lives. And I agreed with him.

To be sure, we need innovations to expand our knowledge and therapies, whether for CF or childhood lymphoma or heart disease or any of the other countless ways in which the human body fails. But we have not effectively used the abilities science has already given us. And we have not made remotely adequate efforts to change that. When we've made a science of performance, however—as we've seen with hand washing, wounded soldiers, child delivery—thousands of lives have been saved. Indeed, the scientific effort to improve performance in medicine—an effort that at present gets only a miniscule portion of scientific budgets—can arguably save more lives in the next decade than bench science, more lives than research on the genome, stem cell therapy, cancer vaccines, and all the other laboratory work we hear about in the news. The stakes could not be higher.

Consider breast cancer. Rates of death from breast cancer have fallen about 25 percent in industrialized countries since 1990. A study of data from a U.S. breast cancer registry recently showed that at least a quarter, and likely more than half, of that decline was due simply to increased use of screening mammography by women. Mammography saves lives by allowing breast cancers to be caught and treated while they're still small, before they can even be felt—and hopefully before they have spread. But the key to its working is that women faithfully get a mammogram once a year. Less often leaves too much time in between for a breast cancer to form, grow, and spread undetected.

So how many women get their mammograms annually? Over five years, one woman in seven does; over ten years, just one in sixteen. The reasons are various. Women themselves are often blamed, but the important underlying factors include how time-consuming, uncomfortable, and difficult it usually is to get a mammogram, how inconvenient the facilities often are, how expensive mammography is for those without insurance coverage, and how rarely reminders are given. The United States government and private foundations spend close to a billion dollars a year on research for discovery of new treatments in breast cancer, but little on innovations to improve the ease of and access to mammography screening.

Nonetheless, studies consistently show that more regular use of this one technology alone would reduce deaths from breast cancer by one-third. This is just one example of what improving performance in medicine could achieve.

I did not completely fathom the full breadth of the possibilities, however, until I considered the practice of medicine in most of the rest of the would—where the best hope for saving lives lies in raising performance, not in expanding genetics research. In 2003, I had just finished my surgical training, and before starting my practice in earnest, I decided to travel as a visiting surgeon to India, my ancestral home. In the course of a two-month tour I worked in a series of six public hospitals across the country—from two-thousand-bed referral centers to rural cottage hospitals and ordinary general hospitals— usually one or two weeks at time.

One of the hospitals I visited was the district hospital that serves Uti, the village my father comes from. Uti is four hundred miles east of Mumbai in the state of Maharashtra and directly north of Karnataka, where I witnessed the polio mop-up. Most of my father's family is still there. He is one of thirteen brothers and sisters. They are farmers. Sugarcane, cotton, and a type of wheat called *jowar* are their cash crops. Drip irrigation has allowed them two crops a year and, along with the money my father sends, that has provided them with a degree of prosperity. Uti has a paved road and electricity. A few houses have running water. Malnutrition is no longer an issue. If the villagers get sick or need a checkup, there is a primary health center with a doctor who comes once a week or so. If they have malaria or a diarrheal illness, he sends them to the cottage hospital in Umarkhed, the small town nearby. Anything more serious and he sends them to the district hospital in Nanded, seventy miles away. This is where my cousin went with his kidney stones.

The Nanded hospital, however, is the lone public hospital serving a district of 1,400 villages like Uti, a population of 2.3 million people. It has five hundred beds, three main operating rooms, and, I found when I visited, just nine general surgeons. (Imagine Kansas with just nine surgeons.) Its two main buildings are four stories high and made of cement and beige stucco. The surgeons arrive each morning to a crush of several hundred people pressing their way into the outpatient clinics. At least two hundred of them are there for the surgery clinic. The inpatient surgical wards are already full. Calls to consult on patients on other services seem never to cease. And the puzzle to me was: How do they do it? How do the surgeons possibly take care of all the hernias and tumors, the appendicitis cases and kidney stones—and manage to sleep, live, survive themselves?

In the clinic one ordinary morning, I accompanied Dr. Ashish Motewar, a general surgeon in his late thirties on duty that day. He had a black Tom Selleck mustache, khaki pants, a blue oxford shirt open at the neck. He did not wear a white coat. His only equipment was a pen, his thin, almost delicate fingers, and his wits.

The clinics at Nanded were like those I found elsewhere in India. They were ovens in the heat of the summer. The paint flaked off the walls in jagged strips. The sinks were stained brown and the faucets didn't work. Each room had a metal desk, some chairs, a whirring ceiling fan, torn squares of blank paper under a stone for writing prescriptions, and at any given moment four, six, sometimes eight patients jockeying for attention. Examinations took place behind a thin rag curtain with gaping tears in it.

In one hour, Motewar saw a sixty-year-old farmer complaining of weight loss, loose bowel movements, and a left-upper-quadrant abdominal mass; a teenage boy with a hot, swollen abscess above his belly button, where he'd been knifed; and three people with right-upper-quadrant pain, two of whom had confirmed gallstones, according to the ultrasound reports they brought with them. A bashful thirty-one-year-old auto-rickshaw driver came in with a walnut-sized tumor growing in his jaw. A turbaned, limping seventy-year-old man dropped his trousers to reveal an aching, incarcerated hernia in his right groin. A father brought his seven-year-old boy in with what turned out to be a rectal prolapse. A silent, scared woman in her thirties undid her sari and uncovered a cancer the size of a child's fist growing into the skin of her breast.

In total, Motewar saw thirty-six patients in three hours that morning. But he was calm despite the chaos. He would smooth down his mustache with his thumb and forefinger and peer silently over his nose at the papers people thrust before him. Then he would speak in a slow and quiet way that made one listen carefully to hear him. He could be brusque at times. But he did what he could to give everyone at least a few moments of individual attention.

With no time for a complete exam, a good history, or explanations, he relied mainly on a quick, finely honed clinical judgment. He sent a few patients out for X-rays and lab tests. The rest he diagnosed on the spot. He summoned a resident to drain the teenager's abscess in an adjacent procedure room. He instructed another resident to schedule the patients with gallstones and the hernia for surgery. A woman with diarrhea and abdominal pain he sent home with medication for worms.

I was especially struck by his treatment of the woman with the eroding breast cancer. Before arriving in India, I had assumed that the complex, expensive treatment such advanced cancers require—chemotherapy, radiation, surgery— would be beyond the system's capabilities and that doctors would simply send patients like her home to die. But the surgeon did no such thing. It was unacceptable. Instead, he admitted the woman directly to the hospital and started her on chemotherapy that same afternoon himself. As a surgeon, I have no idea how to safely administer chemotherapies. In the West, this is something considered so difficult only oncologists know how to do it. But Indian manufacturers produce cheap (often pirated) versions of most drugs, and everywhere I went in India, surgeons had learned how to dose and administer the cyclophosphamide, methotrexate, and fluorouracil themselves, in makeshift treatment rooms of benches and folding chairs. They made compromises out of necessity. They did not monitor blood counts for complications the way we do in richer countries. They gave the drugs through peripheral IVs in patients' arms rather through the expensive central venous lines we use to protect patient's veins from the caustic drugs. But they got the patients through. The same was true for the radiation the patients needed. If they had a working cobalt-60 unit, the kind of radiation therapy unit used in the United States in the 1950s, the surgeons planned and delivered the radiation themselves. If the tumor responded, they then performed surgery. It was textbook treatment devised by other means.

There was, I soon realized, nothing especially exotic about the troubles most people came to the surgeons with, and this in itself was revealing. In the cottage hospital outside my father's village, half the patients were admitted for diseases we do not often see in the West—waterborne diarrhea, tuberculosis, malaria—but it is unusual for them to die from such illnesses. Primary care has improved considerably, and living standards have too. The average life span of Indians has increased from thirty-two years a few decades ago to sixty-five years today. (Two of my aunts were 87 and 92 when I visited and still able to walk their fields. My grandfather finally died at 110 years of age—he fell off a bus and developed a cerebral hemorrhage.) People continue to get cholera and amoebiasis, but they recover. And then they face what we face—gallbladder problems, cancer, hernias, car-crash injuries. The number one cause of death in India is now coronary artery disease, not respiratory infections or diarrheal illness. And most people, even the illiterate, know that medicine can help them survive the "new" afflictions.

The health care system, however, was not built to manage such illnesses—it was designed primarily for infectious disease. The Indian government's annual health care budget of just four dollars per person is woefully little for infectious disease—and impossibly inadequate for something like a heart attack. Improving nutrition, immunization, and sanitation remains a deserved priority. Yet the tide of people needing surgery and other kinds of specialized care does not stop. At least 50 of the 250-some patients seen by the surgeons in Nanded that morning turned out to need an operation. The hospital had operating rooms and staff, however, for only fifteen such operations per day. Everyone else had to wait.

This was the case everywhere I traveled. I spent three weeks as a visiting surgeon at Delhi's All-India Institute of Medical Sciences. Delhi is a spacious and rich city by Indian standards—with broadband, ATMs, malls, and Hondas and Toyotas jostling with the cows and rickshaws on the six-lane asphalt roads. AIIMS is among the country's best-funded, best-staffed public hospitals. Yet even it had a waiting list for essential operations. One day, I accompanied the senior resident charged with supervising the list, kept in a hardbound appointment book. He hated the job. The book recorded the names of four hundred patients awaiting surgery by one of the three faculty surgeons on his team. He was scheduling operations as long as six months in the future. He tried to give patients with cancer the first priority, he told me, but people were constantly accosting him with letters from ministers, employers, and elected officials insisting that he move their cases up in the schedule. By necessity, he accommodated them—and pushed the least connected ever further back in the queue.

The hospital in Nanded did not have anything as formal as a waiting list. The surgeons simply admitted the patients with the most pressing cases and took them to surgery as space and resources became available. As a result, the three surgical wards overflowed with patients. Each ward had sixty metal cots lined up in rows. Some patients had to double up or take a place between the beds on the grimy floor. One day in the men's ward, three beds held an old man recovering from a repair of his strangulated umbilical hernia, a young man who had undergone midnight surgery for a perforated ulcer, and a bespectacled fifty-year-old Sikh waiting, as he had been for the previous week, to have a large inflammatory cyst of the pancreas drained. Across from them, on the floor, a man in his seventies crouched patiently, awaiting resection of his bleeding rectal cancer. Two men nearby shared a bed: a pedestrian who had been hit by a car and a farmer who had been catheterized because of a large stone obstructing his bladder. The surgeons took them as they could, operating through the day and then rotating duty to continue through the night.

In doing this, the surgeons were up against more than just the number of patients. Everywhere, they lacked essential resources. And they lacked the basic systems that we in the West can usually count on to be able to do our jobs.

I am still disgusted by the night I saw a thirty-five-year-old man die from a perfectly treatable lung collapse. He had come to the emergency room at a large city hospital I'd visited. I don't know how long he had waited to be seen. But when I accompanied the surgical resident who was handed his referral slip, we found him sitting up on a bare cot, holding his knees, taking forty breaths a minute, his eyes full of fear. His chest X-ray showed a massive fluid collection in his left chest, obliterating his lung and pushing his heart and trachea to the right. His pulse was rapid. His jugular veins were bulging. He needed immediate chest drainage to let the fluid out and allow his lung to reexpand. Organizing this simple procedure, however, proved to be beyond our capacity.

The resident tried draining the fluid with a needle, but the fluid was infected and too thick for the needle. We needed

to put in a chest tube. But chest tubes—cheap and basic imple-
ments—were out of stock. So the resident handed the man's
brother a prescription for one, and he ran out into the swelter-
ing night to find a medical store that could supply it. Unbeliev-
ably, ten minutes later he came back with one in hand, a 28
French straight chest tube, exactly what we needed. Shortages
of supplies are so common that around any hospital in India
you will find rows of ramshackle stands with vendors selling
everything from medications to pacemakers.

When we got the patient moved to a procedure room to
put in the chest tube, however, no one could locate an instrument set with a knife. The resident ran to find a nurse. And by
this time, I was doing chest compressions. The man was without a pulse or respirations for at least ten minutes before the
resident could finally put a scalpel between his ribs and let the
pus shoot out. It made no difference. The man was dead.

Scarce resources were clearly partly to blame. This was a
hospital of one thousand beds, but it had no chest tubes, no
pulse oximeters, no cardiac monitors, no ability to measure
blood gases. Public hospitals are supposed to be free for patients, but because of inadequate supplies, doctors must routinely ask patients to obtain their own drugs, tubes, tests,
mesh for hernia repairs, staplers, suture material. In one rural
hospital, I met a pale, eighty-year-old man who'd come twenty
miles by bus and on foot to see a doctor about rectal bleeding
from an anal mass, only to be sent right back out because the
hospital had no gloves or lubricating gel to allow the doctor to
provide an examination. A prescription was written, and two
hours later the man hobbled back in, clutching both.

Such problems reflect more than a lack of money, however. In the same hospital where I saw the thirty-five-year-old man die—where basic equipment was lacking, the emergency ward had just two nurses, and filth was everywhere you stepped—there was a brand-new spiral CT scanner and a gorgeous angiography facility that must have cost tens of thousands of dollars to build. More than one doctor told me that it was easier to get a new MRI machine than to maintain basic supplies and hygiene. Such machines have become the symbols of modern medicine, but to view them this way is to misunderstand the nature of medicine's success. Having a machine is not the cure; understanding the ordinary, mundane details that must go right for each particular problem is. India's health system is facing the fundamental and mammoth difficulty of adapting to its population's new and suddenly more complicated range of illnesses. And what's required is rational, reliable organization as much as resources. For surgeons in India, both are in short supply.

This situation is not unique to India, and that is what makes it a core conundrum for our time. Throughout the East, demographics are changing swiftly. In Pakistan, Mongolia, and Papua New Guinea, the average life expectancy has risen to over sixty years. In Sri Lanka, Vietnam, Indonesia, and China, it is more than seventy years. (By contrast, because of AIDS, the expected life span in much of Africa remains under fifty years.) As a result, rates of cancer, traffic accidents, and problems like diabetes and gallstones are exploding worldwide. Cardiac disease has become the globe's leading killer. New laboratory science is not the key to saving lives. The infant science of improving performance—of implementing our existing know-how—is. Nowhere, though, have governments recognized this. A surgeon in much of the world therefore stands on his own, with little more than a pen, his fine fingers, and his wits, to cope with a system that barely works and an ever-growing sea of patients.

These realities are without question demoralizing. The medical community in India has mostly resigned itself to current conditions. All the surgical residents I met hoped to go into the cash-only private sector (where patients with the means increasingly seek care, given the failure of the public system) or abroad when they finished their training—as I think I would, in their shoes. Many attending surgeons were plotting their escape, too. Meanwhile, all live with compromises in the care they give that they cannot bear to tolerate.

Yet, despite the conditions, the surgeons have persisted in developing abilities that were a marvel to witness. I had gone there thinking that, as an American-trained surgeon, I might have a thing or two I could teach them. But the abilities of an average Indian surgeon outstripped those of any Western surgeon I know.

"What is your preferred technique for removing bladder stones?" one surgeon in the city of Nagpur asked me.

"My technique is to call a urologist," I said.

On rounds in Nanded with a staff surgeon one afternoon, I saw patients he'd successfully treated for prostate obstruction, diverticulitis of the colon, a tubercular abscess of the chest, a groin hernia, a thyroid goiter, gallbladder disease, a liver cyst, appendicitis, a staghorn stone in the kidney, and a cancer of the right hand—as well as an infant boy born without an anus in whom he'd done a perfect reconstruction. Using just textbooks and advice from one another, the surgeons at this ordinary district hospital in India had developed an astonishing range of expertise.

What explains this? There was much the surgeons had no control over: the overwhelming flow of patients, the poverty, the lack of supplies. But where they had control—their skills, for example—these doctors sought betterment. They understood themselves to be part of a larger world of medical knowledge and accomplishment. Moreover, they believed they could measure up in it. This was partly, I think, a function of the Nanded surgeons' camaraderie as a group. Each day I was there, the surgeons found time between cases to take a brief late-afternoon break at a café across the street from the hospital. For fifteen or thirty minutes, they drank chai and swapped stories about their cases of the day—what they had done and how. Just this interaction seemed to prod them to aim higher than merely getting through the day. They came to feel they could do anything they set their minds to. Indeed, they believed not only that they were part of the larger world but also that they could contribute to it.

Among the many distressing things I saw in Nanded, one was the incredible numbers of patients with perforated ulcers. In my eight years of surgical training, I had seen only one patient with an ulcer so severe that the stomach's acid had eroded a hole in the intestine. But Nanded is in a part of the country where people eat intensely hot chili peppers, and patients arrived almost nightly with the condition, usually in

severe pain and going into shock after the hours of delay involved in traveling from their villages. The only treatment at
that point is surgical. A surgeon must take the patient to the
operating room urgently, make a slash down the middle of
the abdomen, wash out all the bilious and infected fluid, find
the hole in the duodenum, and repair it. This is a big and traumatic operation, and often these patients were in no condition to survive it. So Motewar did a remarkable thing. He
invented a new operation: a laparoscopic repair of the ulcer-
ous perforation, using quarter-inch incisions and taking an
average of forty-five minutes. When I later told colleagues at
home about the operation, they were incredulous. It did not
seem possible.

Motewar, however, had mulled over the ulcer problem
off and on for years and became convinced he could devise a
better treatment. His department was able to obtain some
older laparoscopic equipment inexpensively. An assistant was
made personally responsible for keeping it clean and in working order. And over time, Motewar carefully worked out his
technique. I saw him do the operation, and it was elegant and
swift. He even did a randomized trial, which he presented at a
conference and which revealed the operation to have fewer
complications and a far more rapid recovery than the standard
procedure. In that remote, dust-covered town in Maharashtra,
Motewar and his colleagues had become among the most pro-
ficient ulcer surgeons in the world.

True success in medicine is not easy. It requires will, attention to detail, and creativity. But the lesson I took from India was that it is possible anywhere and by anyone. I can
imagine few places with more difficult conditions. Yet aston-

ishing successes could be found. And each one began, I noticed, remarkably simply: with a readiness to recognize problems and a determination to remedy them.

Arriving at meaningful solutions is an inevitably slow and difficult process. Nonetheless, what I saw was: better is possible. It does not take genius. It takes diligence. It takes moral clarity. It takes ingenuity. And above all, it takes a willingness to try.

THERE WAS A one-year-old boy I saw brought into the teeming Nanded surgery clinic by his parents, their faces wearing that distressing look of fear, helplessness, and fervent hope I'd come to recognize in poor, overcrowded hospitals. The child lay in the cradle of his mother's arms disturbingly quiet, his eyes open but without interest or reaction. His breathing was steady and unlabored yet unnaturally fast—as if a pump inside him were set at the wrong speed. The mother described repeated bouts of frighteningly violent vomiting—the emesis could burst out of him across a table. A doctor in the pediatric clinic had noted his head to be enlarged, with a circumference distinctly out of proportion to his small body, and made a provisional diagnosis that was confirmed on a skull X-ray: the boy had a severe hydrocephalus—a congenital disease in which the normal drainage of the brain is blocked. The cerebral fluid slowly accumulates, gradually expanding the skull but also compressing the brain to relieve the pressure. Unless surgery is performed to provide a new route out of the brain and skull for the fluid, the resulting brain damage becomes severe, advancing from vomiting to visual loss to sleepiness, coma, and finally death. But if surgery were successfully done, the child could live completely normally. The pediatricians had therefore sent the child and his parents to the surgery clinic.

The surgery department had no neurosurgeon, though. Nor did it have the equipment a neurosurgeon would need—no drill to burr a hole through the skull, no shunt device with its sterile, one-way-flow tubing to channel the fluid out of the brain, under the skin, and down into the abdominal cavity. The surgeons did not want to just let the child die, however. They gave the father instructions about the sort of device his son needed, and he managed to find a facsimile of one in the local market for 1,500 rupees (about thirty dollars). It was not perfect—the tubing was too long and it wasn't sterile. But P. T. Jamdade, the chief of surgery, agreed to take the case.

The child was brought to the operating room the next day, my last in Nanded, and I watched the surgical team perform. The tubing was trimmed to size and put in a steam autoclave. The anesthetist put the boy to sleep with an injection of ketamine, a cheap and effective anesthetic. A nurse shaved the hair from the right side of his head with a razor and cleansed his skin from head to hips with an iodine antiseptic. A surgical resident laid sterile cloth drapes down to frame the operative field. On a little tray under a lone operating light, a nurse lined up the surgical instruments—silvery, gleaming, and, it seemed to me, wholly inadequate to the task. Jamdade had little more to work with than I would use to sew a minor laceration closed. But he took the scalpel and made a one-inch incision through the skin and thin muscle an inch above the boy's ear. He took a hemostat—an ordinary scissors-shaped metal clamp that surgeons normally use to grasp a small blood vessel or a suture thread—and began slowly grinding its tip into the child's exposed white skull.

At first, nothing happened. The tip kept sliding off the hard, bony surface. But it began to find purchase, and over the next fifteen painstaking minutes he ground and scraped until a tiny hole through the skull appeared. He worked to widen the aperture, taking care not to slip and puncture the now exposed brain. When the opening was large enough, he slid an end of the tubing through into the space between the brain and the skull. He took the other end of the tubing and snaked it under the skin of the neck and chest down to the abdomen. Before popping the tubing into the open space of the abdominal cavity, though, he stopped momentarily to watch the fluid of the brain flowing out of its new channel. It was clear and lovely, like water. Like perfection. He had not given up. And as a result, at least this one child would live.

Afterword: Suggestions for Becoming a Positive Deviant

In October 2003, upon my return from India, I officially began my life as a general and endocrine surgeon in Boston. Mondays, I saw patients in a third-floor surgical clinic at my hospital. Tuesdays and some weekends, I took emergency call. Wednesdays, I saw patients at an outpatient clinic across the street from Fenway Park. Thursdays and Fridays, I spent in the operating room doing surgery. It has proved to be an orderly life, and I am grateful for that. Nonetheless, there was much I wasn't prepared for, including how small one's place in the world inevitably proves to be. Most of us, most of the time, are far removed from planning a polio mop-up for 4.2 million children in southern India or inventing new ways to save the lives of frontline soldiers. Our enterprise is more modest. In my clinic on a Monday afternoon, I need to think about Mrs. X and her gallstones; Mr. Y and his painful hernia; Ms. Z and her breast lump. Medicine is retail. We can tend to only one person at a time.

No doctor wants to believe that he or she is a bit player, though. After all, doctors are given the power to prescribe more than 6,600 potentially dangerous drugs. We are permitted to open human beings up like melons. Soon we will even be allowed to manipulate their DNA. People depend on us personally for their lives. And yet, as a doctor each of us is just one of 819,000 physicians and surgeons in this country tasked with helping people live lives as long and healthy as possible. And even that overestimates the size of our contributions. In on this work are also 2.4 million nurses, 388,000 medical assistants, 232,000 pharmacists, 294,000 lab technicians, 121,000 paramedics, 94,000 respiratory therapists, 85,000 nutritionists.

It can be hard not to feel that one is just a white-coated cog in a machine—an extraordinarily successful machine, but a machine nonetheless. How could it be otherwise? The average American can expect to live at least seventy-eight years. But reaching, and surpassing, that age depends more on this system of millions of people than on any one individual within it. None of us is irreplaceable. So not surprisingly, in this work one begins to wonder: How do I really matter?

I get to lecture to the students at our medical school on occasion. For one lecture, I decided to try to figure out an answer to this question, both for them and for myself. I came up with five—five suggestions for how one might make a worthy difference, for how one might become, in other words, a positive deviant. This is what I told them.

⋆   ⋆   ⋆

MY FIRST SUGGESTION came from a favorite essay by Paul Auster: *Ask an unscripted question*. Ours is a job of talking to strangers. Why not learn something about them?

On the surface, this seems easy enough. Then your new patient arrives. You still have three others to see and two pages to return, and the hour is getting late. In that instant, all you want is to proceed with the matter at hand. Where's the pain, the lump, whatever the trouble is? How long has it been there? Does anything make it better or worse? What are the person's past medical problems? Everyone knows the drill.

But consider, at an appropriate point, taking a moment with your patient. Make yourself ask an unscripted question: "Where did you grow up?" Or: "What made you move to Boston?" Even: "Did you watch last night's Red Sox game?" You don't have to come up with a deep or important question, just one that lets you make a human connection. Some people won't be interested in making that connection. They'll just want you to look at the lump. That's OK. In that case, look at the lump. Do your job.

You will find, however, that many respond—because they're polite, or friendly, or perhaps in need of human contact. When this happens, try seeing if you can keep the conversation going for more than two sentences. Listen. Make note of what you learn. This is not a forty-six-year-old male with a right inguinal hernia. This is a forty-six-year-old former mortician who hated the funeral business with a right inguinal hernia.

One can of course do this with people other than patients. So ask a random question of the medical assistant who checks their vitals, a nurse you run into on rounds. It's not that making this connection necessarily helps anyone. But you start to remember the people you see, instead of letting them all blur together. And sometimes you discover the unexpected. I learned, for instance, that an elderly Pakistani phlebotomist I saw every day during my residency had been a general surgeon in Karachi for twenty years but emigrated for the sake of his children's education. I found out that a quiet, carefully buttoned-down nurse I work with had once dated Jimi Hendrix.

If you ask a question, the machine begins to feel less like a machine.

MY SECOND SUGGESTION was: *Don't complain.* To be sure, a doctor has plenty to carp about: predawn pages, pointless paperwork, computer system crashes, a new problem popping up at six o'clock on a Friday night. We all know what it feels like to be tired and beaten down. Yet nothing in medicine is more dispiriting than hearing doctors complain.

Recently, I joined a group of surgeons and nurses having lunch in the hospital cafeteria. The banter started off cheerily enough. First we chatted about a patient one of the surgeons had seen (a man with a tumor the size of his head growing out of his back), then about the two cans of Diet Vanilla Coke we watched one of the nurses consume. (The Coca-Cola Company had discontinued the flavor—such as it is—but she had hoarded enough to keep herself in supply.) Next, however, a surgeon told a bitter tale of being called to the emergency department at 2:00 A.M. the previous Sunday to see a woman with a severely infected gallbladder. He had advised that she would best be treated with antibiotics, fluids, admission to the hospital, and a delay in surgery until the inflammation had subsided, only to have the emergency physician tell her that such a plan was dangerous and she should be operated upon right away. The emergency physician was wrong, the surgeon said. Worse, he had not had the common courtesy to pick up the phone and discuss his concerns before speaking to the patient. When the surgeon confronted him later, he was not in the least apologetic. The story unleashed from the others a raft of similar tales of unprofessional behavior. And when lunch was over, we all returned to our operating rooms and hospital wards feeling angry and sorry for ourselves.

Medicine is a trying profession, but less because of the difficulties of disease than because of the difficulties of having to work with other human beings under circumstances only partly in one's control. Ours is a team sport, but with two key differences from the kinds with lighted scoreboards: the stakes are people's lives and we have no coaches. The latter is no minor matter. Doctors are expected to coach themselves. We have no one but ourselves to lift us through the struggles. But we're not good at it. Wherever doctors gather—in meeting rooms, in conference halls, in hospital cafeterias—the natural pull of conversational gravity is toward the litany of woes all around us.

But resist it. It's boring, it doesn't solve anything, and it will get you down. You don't have to be sunny about everything. Just be prepared with something else to discuss: an idea you read about, an interesting problem you came across—

even the weather if that's all you've got. See if you can keep the conversation going.

MY THIRD ANSWER for becoming a positive deviant: *Count something*. Regardless of what one ultimately does in medicine—or outside medicine, for that matter—one should be a scientist in this world. In the simplest terms, this means one should count something. The laboratory researcher may count the number of tumor cells in a petri dish that have a particular gene defect. Likewise, the clinician might count the number of patients who develop a particular complication from treatment—or just how many are actually seen on time and how many are made to wait. It doesn't really matter what you count. You don't need a research grant. The only requirement is that what you count should be interesting to you.

When I was a resident I began counting how often our surgical patients ended up with an instrument or sponge forgotten inside them. It didn't happen often: about one in fifteen thousand operations, I discovered. But when it did, serious injury could result. One patient had a thirteen-inch retractor left in him that tore into his bowel and bladder. Another had a small sponge left in his brain that caused an abscess and a permanent seizure disorder.

Then I counted how often such mistakes occurred because the nurses hadn't counted all the sponges as they were supposed to or because the doctors had ignored nurses' warnings that an item was missing. It turned out to be hardly ever. Eventually I got a little more sophisticated and compared patients who had objects left inside them with those who didn't.

I found that the mishaps predominantly occurred in patients undergoing emergency operations or procedures that revealed the unexpected—such as a cancer when the surgeon had anticipated only appendicitis.

The numbers began to make sense. If nurses have to track fifty sponges and a couple of hundred instruments during an operation—already a tricky thing to do—it is understandably much harder under urgent circumstances or when unexpected changes require bringing in lots more equipment. Our usual approach of punishing people for failures wasn't going to eliminate the problem, I realized. Only a technological solution would—and I soon found myself working with some colleagues to come up with a device that could automate the tracking of sponges and instruments.

If you count something you find interesting, you will learn something interesting.

MY FOURTH SUGGESTION was: *Write something*. I do not mean this to be an intimidating suggestion. It makes no difference whether you write five paragraphs for a blog, a paper for a professional journal, or a poem for a reading group. Just write. What you write need not achieve perfection. It need only add some small observation about your world.

You should not underestimate the effect of your contribution, however modest. As Lewis Thomas once pointed out, quoting the physicist John Ziman, "The invention of a mechanism for the systematic publication of 'fragments' of scientific work may well have been the key event in the history of modern science." By soliciting modest contributions from the many, we have produced a store of collective know-how with far greater power than any individual could have achieved. And this is as true outside science as inside.

You should also not underestimate the power of the act of writing itself. I did not write until I became a doctor. But once I became a doctor, I found I needed to write. For all its complexity, medicine is more physically than intellectually taxing. Because medicine is a retail enterprise, because doctors provide their services to one person after another, it can be a grind. You can lose your larger sense of purpose. But writing lets you step back and think through a problem. Even the angriest rant forces the writer to achieve a degree of thoughtfulness.

Most of all, by offering your reflections to an audience, even a small one, you make yourself part of a larger world. Put a few thoughts on a topic in just a newsletter, and you find yourself wondering nervously: Will people notice it? What will they think? Did I say something dumb? An audience is a community. The published word is a declaration of membership in that community and also of a willingness to contribute something meaningful to it.

So choose your audience. Write something.

MY SUGGESTION NUMBER five, my final suggestion for a life in medicine, was: *Change*. In medicine, just as in anything else people do, individuals respond to new ideas in one of three ways. A few become early adopters, as the business types call them. Most become late adopters. And some remain persistent skeptics who never stop resisting. A doctor may have good reasons to take any of these stances. When Jonas Salk tried out his new polio vaccine on over 400,000 children, when a battlefield surgeon first shipped a soldier to Landstuhl with the bleeding stopped but his abdomen open and the operation unfinished, when Warren Warwick began putting more feeding tubes into CF children—who was to say whether these were truly good ideas? Medicine has seen plenty of bad ones. Frontal lobotomies were once performed for the control of chronic pain. The anti-inflammatory medication Vioxx turned out to cause heart attacks. Viagra, it was recently discovered, may cause partial vision loss.

Nonetheless, make yourself an early adopter. Look for the opportunity to change. I am not saying you should embrace every new trend that comes along. But be willing to recognize the inadequacies in what you do and to seek out solutions. As successful as medicine is, it remains replete with uncertainties and failure. This is what makes it human, at times painful, and also so worthwhile.

The choices a doctor makes are necessarily imperfect but they alter people's lives. Because of that reality, it often seems safest to do what everyone else is doing—to be just another white-coated cog in the machine. But a doctor must not let that happen—nor should anyone who takes on risk and responsibility in society.

So find something new to try, something to change. Count how often you succeed and how often you fail. Write about it. Ask people what they think. See if you can keep the conversation going.

Notes on Sources

On Washing Hands

14 The U.S. Centers for Disease Control's "Guideline for Hand Hygiene in Health-Care Settings," by J. M. Boyce and D. Pittet, was published in the *Morbidity and Mortality Weekly Report*, October 25, 2002, pp. 1–44. It can also be found at www.cdc.gov.

15 Sherwin Nuland tells the tale of Semmelweis in *The Doctors' Plague: Germs, Childbed Fever, and the Strange Story of Ignac Semmelweis* (New York: Norton, 2003).

24 The article that Jon Lloyd came across about the Sternins' approach to reducing starvation in Vietnam was D. Dorsey's "Positive Deviant," in *Fast Company*, November 2000, p. 284. More about positive deviance can be found at www.positivedeviance.org.

THE MOP-UP

29   The definition of diligence is from the *Random House Unabridged Dictionary* (New York: Random House, 2006).

31   For an overview of WHO's eradication efforts, see G. Williams, "WHO: The Days of the Mass Campaigns," *World Health Forum* 9 (1988): 7–23.

32   A campaign against guinea worm disease, led by the Carter Center and financed by the CDC, WHO, and the Gates Foundation, is the only global eradication program now under way besides the one against polio (see www.cartercenter.org). As with the polio effort, there remains great hope. The parasitic worm was once endemic in Africa and Asia and caused some three to ten million infections per year. (The worms grow to three feet in length in the abdomen and then emerge slowly and painfully through the skin, incapacitating victims for two months or longer.) The worm has now been confined to a dozen African countries and only ten thousand infections occurred in 2005. Success again has depended on incredible attention to surveillance and follow-through in prevention.

50   The Web site www.polioeradication.org has up-to-date information on the current number of polio cases and maps with the locations of outbreaks.

CASUALTIES OF WAR

51   The U.S. Department of Defense's weekly update on American military casualties can be found at http://www.defenselink.mil/news/casualty.pdf.

52   The study that first examined the relationship between homicide rates and medical care is A. R. Harris, S. H. Thomas, G. A. Fisher, and D. J. Hirsch, "Murder and Medicine: The Lethality

of Criminal Assault, 1960–1999," *Homicide Studies* 6 (2002): 128–66.

52 The source for the historical casualty numbers is U.S. Department of Defense, "Principal Wars in which the United States Participated: U.S. Military Personnel Serving and Casualties," 2004 (http://web1.whs.osd.mil/mmid/casualty/WCPRINCIPAL .pdf). Some experts have argued that the DoD online data is inaccurate, because of changing definitions of who is wounded (see J. B. Holcomb, L. G. Stansbury, H. R. Champion, C. Wade, and R. F. Bellamy, *Journal of Trauma* 60 [2006]: 397–401). If figures are restricted to casualties known to have required at least some hospital care, the lethality rate for the American war wounded was 23 percent in World War II (using army-only data), 23 percent in the Korean War, and anywhere from 16 to 24 percent in the Vietnam War (the definitions for Vietnam remain contentious to this day). (These data are from G. Beebe and M. E. DeBakey, *Battle Casualties: Incidence, Mortality, and Logistic Considerations* [Springfield: Charles C. Thomas, 1952]; F. A. Reister, *Battle Casualties and Medical Statistics: U.S. Army Experience in Korea* [Washington: Department of the Army, 1973]; R. F. Bellamy, "Why Is Marine Combat Mortality Less Than That of the Army?" *Military Medicine* 165 [2000]: 362–67.) Using this definition of wounded, lethality of war wounds for American troops in the Persian Gulf War was 24 percent; in the current wars in Iraq and Afghanistan it has been no higher than 12 percent.

57 For more on Ronald Bellamy's concept of the "Golden Five Minutes," see his chapter on combat trauma in his *Textbook of Military Medicine: Anesthesia and Pre-Operative Care of the Combat Casualty* (Washington: Department of the Army, Office of the Surgeon General, Borden Institute, 1994), pp. 1–42.

Naked

77   The U.K. standards on physical examination etiquette are described in the General Medical Council's report *Intimate Examinations* (London: General Medical Council Standards Committee, December 2001) and in the Royal College of Obstetricians and Gynaecologists' *Gynaecological Examinations: Guidelines for Specialist Practice* (London: Royal College of Obstetricians and Gynaecologists, July 2002).

78   I relied on three reports in particular in considering the etiquette of American examinations: The Ad Hoc Committee on Physician Impairment's *Report on Sexual Boundary Issues* (Dallas: Federation of State Medical Boards of the United States, April 1996); C. E. Dehlendorf and S. M. Wolfe, "Physicians Disciplined for Sex-Related Offenses," *JAMA* 279 (1998): 1883–88; and J. A. Enbom and C. D. Thomas, "Evaluation of Sexual Misconduct Complaints: The Oregon Board of Medical Examiners, 1991 to 1995," *American Journal of Obstetrics and Gynecology* 176 (1997): 1340–48.

79   Data on patient-initiated sexual behavior toward medical students comes from a report by H. M. Schulte and J. Kay in *Academic Medicine* 69 (1995): 842–46.

What Doctors Owe

87   Much of the detail on the American medical malpractice system comes from research by my colleagues David Studdert, Michelle Mello, and Troy Brennan of the Harvard School of Public Health. See, for example, D. M. Studdert et al., "Negligent Care and Malpractice Claiming Behavior in Utah and Colorado," *Medical Care* 38 (2000): 250–60, and D. M. Studdert et al., "Claims, Errors, and Compensation Payments in Medical

Malpractice Litigation," *New England Journal of Medicine* 354 (2006): 2024–33. Two excellent reviews of what we know about the American malpractice system are D. M. Studdert, M. M. Mello, T. A. Brennan, "Medical Malpractice," *New England Journal of Medicine* 350 (2004): 283–92 (that's a short one), and Tom Baker's *The Medical Malpractice Myth* (Chicago: University of Chicago Press, 2005) (that's a longer one).

108 For more on the National Vaccine Injury Compensation program, see D. Ridgway's description in the *Journal of Health Politics, Policy, and Law* 24 (1999): 59–90, and also the program's Web site, www.hrsa.gov/osp/vicp/.

109 The New Zealand malpractice system is detailed by M. Bismark and R. Paterson in "No-Fault Compensation in New Zealand," *Health Affairs* 25 (2000): 278–83.

PIECEWORK

116 William Hsiao outlined his evaluation of the relative amount of work involved in the different tasks physicians do—the relative value scale—in two principal articles: W. Hsiao et al., "Resource-Based Relative Values: An Overview," *JAMA* 260 (1988): 2347–53, and W. Hsiao et al., "Measurement and Analysis of Intraservice Work," *JAMA* 260 (1988): 2361–70.

120 William Weeks's studies of how much physicians work and earn and the comparison with other professions were published in W. Weeks and A. Wallace, "Time and Money: A Retrospective Evaluation of the Inputs, Outputs, Efficiency, and Incomes of Physicians," *Archives of Internal Medicine* 163 (2003): 944–48, and W. Weeks and A. Wallace, "The More Things Change: Revisiting a Comparison of Educational Costs and Incomes of Physicians and Other Professionals," *Academic Medicine* 77 (2002): 312–19.

126 The amount of money currently spent on health care in the United States is tracked by the government, and the figures are available from the Medicare Web site: www.cms.hhs.gov/NationalHealthExpendData/.

128 Information on doctors' incomes relative to average workers' incomes was found in Derek Bok's fascinating book *The Cost of Talent* (New York: Free Press, 1993) and in data from the Bertelsmann Foundation's International Reform Monitor (see www.reformmonitor.org).

128 Evidence on the health and financial consequences of lacking insurance can be found in Jack Hadley's "Sicker and Poorer," *Medical Care Research and Review* 60 (2003): 3S–75S.

THE DOCTORS OF THE DEATH CHAMBER

130 The full opinion of United States District Judge Jeremy Fogel in the case of *Michael Angelo Morales v. Roderick Q. Hickman* is a riveting and surprisingly readable document (No. C 06 219 JF; District Court, Northern District of California: February 14, 2006). Also see the appeals court's ruling specifying what participating anesthesiologists would be required to do to ensure a rapid, painless death for an inmate (*Michael Angelo Morales v. Roderick Q. Hickman*, No. CV 06 00926 JF; U.S. 9th Circuit of Appeals: February 20, 2006).

132 The history of lethal injection and other execution methods is told in Stephen Trombley's fine book *The Execution Protocol: Inside America's Capital Punishment Industry* (New York: Crown, 1992). Similarly intriguing is Ivan Solotaroff's *The Last Face You'll Ever See: The Private Life of the American Death Penalty* (New York: HarperCollins, 2001).

134 Ethics codes for participation in executions by different medical professions can be found as follows: The American Medical

Association's position was published in *JAMA* 270 (1993): 365–68, and is available on the www.ama-assn.org Web site. The Society of Correctional Physicians puts its ethics code online at http://www.corrdocs.org/about/ethics.html. The American Nursing Association's position statement on nurses' participation in capital punishment is available at http://nursingworld .org/readroom/position/ethics/prtetcptl.htm. The American Pharmaceutical Association's current policies are found in its "policies related to the practice environment and quality of worklife issues," available at www.aphanet.org.

136   Current data on death penalty cases is available from the Death Penalty Information Center Execution Database at http:// www.deathpenaltyinfo.org/executions.php.

137   The seminal study on physician participation in U.S. executions is *Breach of Trust* (Philadelphia: American College of Physicians and Physicians for Human Rights, 1994).

141   The survey I cite on the level of physician awareness of ethics guidelines on participation in executions was published by N. J. Farber et al. in *Annals of Internal Medicine* 135 (2001): 884–88.

152   On the U.S. government's recent willingness to use medical skills against individuals for state purposes, see Stephen Miles's *Oath Betrayed: Torture, Medical Complicity, and the War on Terror* (New York: Random House, 2006).

ON FIGHTING

159   Watson Bowes Jr.'s study of aggressively resuscitating premature infants was published with his colleagues M. Halgrimson and M. A. Simmons in the *Journal of Reproductive Medicine* 23 (1979): 245.

THE SCORE

172 Information on the normal anatomy, physiology, and process of labor, as well as the abnormalities that can occur, is taken from F. G. Cunningham et al., eds., *Williams Obstetrics*, 22nd ed. (New York: McGraw-Hill, 2005).

176 The details of the history of obstetrical techniques and complications are from numerous sources, in particular: J. Drife, "The Start of Life: A History of Obstetrics," *Postgraduate Medical Journal* 78 (2002): 311–15; R. W. Wertz and D. C. Wertz, *Lying-In: A History of Childbirth in America* (New Haven: Yale University Press, 1989); and D. Trolle, *The History of Caesarean Section* (Copenhagen: University Library, 1982).

179 For more data on the modern experience of childbirth, including on how commonly laboring mothers turn to medical interventions such as electronic monitors, epidurals, and labor-stimulating medication, an excellent source is E. R. Declercq et al., *Listening to Mothers: Report of the First National U.S. Survey of Women's Childbearing Experiences* (New York: Maternity Center Association, 2002).

184 Historical data on perinatal mortality for mothers and newborns are from the U.S. Centers for Disease Control.

185 Shortly after Virginia Apgar's death, her friend and colleague L. Stanley James published his eulogy, "Fond Memories of Virginia Apgar," in *Pediatrics* 55 (1975): 1–4. Another key source of information on her life is A. A. Skolnick, "Apgar Quartet Plays Perinatologist's Instruments," *JAMA* 276 (1996): 1939–40. An excellent review of the development and importance of her score is M. Finster and M. Wood, "The Apgar Score Has Survived the Test of Time," *Anesthesiology* 102 (2005): 855–57.

188 The 1979 ranking of specialties' use of randomized trials was undertaken by the father of evidence-based medicine, Archie

L. Cochrane, in his article "1931–1971: A Critical Review with Particular Reference to the Medical Profession," in G. Teeling-Smith and N. Wells, eds., *Medicines for the Year 2000* (London: Office of Health Economics, 1979).

190 Watson Bowes Jr. and V. L. Katz published a 1994 review of studies of forceps deliveries, including a comparison with Cesarean sections, entitled "Operative Vaginal Delivery," in *Current Problems in Obstetrics, Gynecology, and Fertility* 17 (1994): 86. A 1979 Australian study, for example, compared 296 forceps deliveries with 101 Cesarean sections and 207 spontaneous vaginal deliveries. The children did equally well, including on IQ and motor tests at age five (W. G. McBride et al., "Method of Delivery and Developmental Outcome at Five Years of Age," *Medical Journal of Australia* 1, no. 8 [1979]: 301–4). A few studies showed some practitioners could achieve better results with forceps. A 1990 study, for example, compared 358 forceps deliveries with 486 Cesarean sections at UCLA and found that, while the infants had no differences in their Apgar scores or rates of birth trauma, the mothers had fewer complications and less blood loss with forceps (R. A. Bashore, W. H. Phillips Jr., C. R. Brinkman III, "A Comparison of the Morbidity of Midforceps and Cesarean Delivery," *American Journal of Obstetrics & Gynecology* 162, no. 6 [1990]: 1428–34).

197 A definitive review of the benefit and risks of elective Cesarean sections for pregnant mothers at full term was published in March 2006 by the National Institutes of Health and is available from their Web site, www.nih.gov. It is entitled "National Institutes of Health State-of-the-Science Conference Statement: Cesarean Delivery on Maternal Request." See also H. Minkoff and F. A. Chervenak, "Elective Primary Cesarean Delivery," *New England Journal of Medicine* 348 (2003): 946–50.

THE BELL CURVE

206   Information on bell curves in hernia repair is from data collected for a Veterans Administration study: R. J. Fitzgibbons et al., "Watchful Waiting vs. Repair of Inguinal Hernia in Minimally Symptomatic Men," *JAMA* 295 (2006): 285–92. Risk-adjusted neonatal ICU outcomes are from the Vermont Oxford Network Database (*Health Affairs* 23 [2004]: 89). In vitro fertilization center outcomes are available from the CDC at www.cdc.gov/ART.

208   An intriguing examination of the U.S. government's ill-fated Death List is S. T. Mennemeyer, M. A. Morrisey, and L. Z. Howard's "Death and Reputation: How Consumers Acted upon HCFA Mortality Information," *Inquiry* 34 (1997): 117–28.

209   For more on the superior performance of LeRoy Matthews's CF treatment program in Cleveland, see W. J. Warwick, "Cystic Fibrosis: Nature and Prognosis," *Minnesota Medicine* 50 (1967): 1049–53; L. W. Matthews and C. F. Doershuk, "Management-Comprehensive Treatment of Cystic Fibrosis," *Minnesota Medicine* 52 (1969): 1506–14; and American Thoracic Society, "The Treatment of Cystic Fibrosis: A Statement by the Committee on Therapy," *American Review of Respiratory Disease* 97 (1968): 730–34.

211   No one has done more to tease apart the relative contributions of genetics, sociodemographics, and differences in treatment programs in cystic fibrosis than Michael S. Schecter, a pediatric pulmonologist and CF expert at Hasbro Children's Hospital, Providence, Rhode Island. See in particular his article "Non-Genetic Influences on CF Lung Disease: The Role of Socio-demographic Characteristics, Environmental Exposures, and Healthcare Interventions," *Pediatric Pulmonology* 26 (2004): 82–85.

For Performance

237 Data on the inadequacies of mammography screening in the United States come from two articles: K. A. Phillips et al., "Factors Associated with Women's Adherence to Mammography Screening Guidelines," *Health Services Research* 33 (1998): 29–53, and K. Blanchard et al., "Mammographic Screening: Patterns of Use and Estimated Impact on Breast Carcinoma Survival," *Cancer* 101 (2005): 495–507.

242 For more on the increasing longevity of much of the world's population and the resulting shift in patterns of disease, see the World Health Organization's *The World Health Report 1999: Making a Difference* (Geneva: World Health Organization, 1999), and J. A. Salomon and C. J. L. Murray, "The Epidemiologic Transition Revisited: Compositional Models for Causes of Death by Age and Sex," *Population and Development Review* 28 (2002): 205–28.

Afterword: Suggestions for Becoming a Positive Deviant

251 That favorite essay of Paul Auster's is "Gotham Handbook," in *Collected Prose* (New York: Picador, 2003), and I owe to it not only the first rule but the structure of this chapter—and an understanding of the importance of talking about the weather.

255 The study of forgotten surgical tools was published in the *New England Journal of Medicine* 348 (2003): 229–35.

255 Lewis Thomas's quoting of John Ziman is in his essay "On Societies as Organisms," in *Lives of a Cell* (New York: Penguin, 1974).

Acknowledgments

Among several people indispensable to this book, my research assistant, Ami Karlage, comes foremost. She is whip smart and insanely resourceful and had better ways she could have spent three years of her life. But she helped research every chapter here and was essential to my making this book as rich and accurate as possible.

If Ami gave in breadth, my wife, Kathleen Hobson, gave in depth. She has made my successes and failures her own. She has pushed and encouraged this book and talked me through my uncertainties and confusions about it. And she made writing it possible alongside everything else in our life together.

I also owe particular thanks to my friends Burkhard Bilger, Henry Finder, Malcolm Gladwell, and David Segal. Four of the smartest people I know, they gave generously of their time and energy in thinking through my ideas for this book. I am lucky to have Henry as my editor at the *New Yorker*, as well—he not only midwifed the five chapters here that had begun as magazine pieces but has been my closest mentor for my writing career. The other essential person for that career has been David Remnick, who has let me continue as a *New Yorker* staff writer despite having to accommodate the demands of my surgical career. The opportunity to write for the magazine means more to me than I can possibly say.

The great Sara Bershtel of Metropolitan Books was my editor for *Better*, as she was for *Complications*. And she has proved to be the kind of book editor one hears no longer exists: she cares deeply about writing and ideas, and she edits. Her colleague Riva Hocherman also offered invaluable suggestions. Both made this book better in every way.

My longtime friend Tina Bennett has also been, for the past seven years, my agent, an arrangement that would ordinarily be considered dicey. But her judgment is impeccable. She is indefatigable. And she has proved as wise and loyal in her advocacy as an agent as she has in her devotion as a friend.

Several of the chapters began as articles I had written for the *New England Journal of Medicine*, and I am grateful to Debra Malina, Greg Curfman, Steve Morrissey, and Jeff Drazen of the *Journal* for their support, advice, and encouragement.

Finishing this book would not have been possible without the understanding and support of my surgical colleagues, in particular: Michael Zinner, the chief of surgery at Brigham and Women's Hospital; Stan Ashley, the chief of general surgery at Harvard Vanguard Medical Associates; and Francis

"Chip" Moore, my surgical partner. Thank you also to Susan Cramer, Shilpa Rao, and Katy Thompson of Brigham and Women's Hospital, Arnie Epstein of the Harvard School of Public Health, and John Sterling of Henry Holt Publishing.

Finally, I want to give my deep thanks to the patients and colleagues who appear, named and unnamed, in this book. They gave me permission to try to tell their stories, and that is the most generous and vital gift of all.

About the Author

ATUL GAWANDE, a 2006 MacArthur Fellow, is a general surgeon at the Brigham and Women's Hospital in Boston, a staff
writer for *The New Yorker*, an assistant professor at Harvard
Medical School and the Harvard School of Public Health, and
a frequent contributor to *The New England Journal of Medicine*.
His first book, *Complications: A Surgeon's Notes on an Imperfect
Science*, was a *New York Times* bestseller and a finalist for the
2002 National Book Award. Gawande lives with his wife and
three children in Newton, Massachusetts.